Cardiac Arrhythmias: From Mechanisms to Management

Cardiac Arrhythmias: From Mechanisms to Management

Editor: Rowan Cook

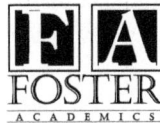

FOSTER
ACADEMICS

www.fosteracademics.com

www.fosteracademics.com

FA
FOSTER
ACADEMICS

Cataloging-in-Publication Data

Cardiac arrhythmias : from mechanisms to management / edited by Rowan Cook.
    p. cm.
Includes bibliographical references and index.
ISBN 978-1-63242-605-5
1. Arrhythmia. 2. Heart--Diseases--Treatment. 3. Heart beat.
4. Cardiology. I. Cook, Rowan.
RC685.A65 C37 2019
616.128--dc23

Foster Academics,
118-35 Queens Blvd., Suite 400,
Forest Hills, NY 11375, USA

ISBN 978-1-63242-605-5 (Hardback)

Contents

Preface VII

Chapter 1   **Breijo Electrocardiographic Pattern**..1
              Francisco R. Breijo-Márquez

Chapter 2   **Histopathological Change Following Cox-Maze IV Procedure
              for Atrial Fibrillation** 16
              Takashi Murashita

Chapter 3   **Drug Abuse-Induced Cardiac Arrhythmias: Mechanisms
              and Management**...29
              Sana Ouali, Omar Guermazi, Fatma Guermazi, Manel Ben Halima,
              Selim Boudiche, Nadim Khedher, Fathia Meghaieth,
              Abdeljalil Farhati, Noureddine Larbi and Mohamed Sami Mourali

Chapter 4   **Endocardial Approach for Substrate Ablation in Brugada Syndrome**......................46
              Pablo E. Tauber, Virginia Mansilla, Pedro Brugada, Sara S. Sánchez,
              Stella M. Honoré, Marcelo Elizari, Sergio Chain Molina,
              Felix A. Albano, Ricardo R. Corbalán, Federico Figueroa Castellanos
              and Damian Alzugaray Bioeng

Chapter 5   **Atrial Flutter: Diagnosis and Management Strategies** 69
              Hamid Reza Bonakdar

Chapter 6   **Brugada Type 1 Pattern and Risk Stratification for Sudden
              Death: Does the Key Hide in the ECG Analysis?**...88
              Antoine Deliniere, Francis Bessiere, Adrien Moreau, Alexandre Janin,
              Gilles Millat and Philippe Chevalier

Chapter 7   **Gene Polymorphisms Associated with Atrial Fibrillation** 106
              Nevra Alkanli, Arzu Ay and Suleyman Serdar Alkanli

Chapter 8   **Idiopathic Ventricular Arrhythmias** 126
              Takumi Yamada

Chapter 9   **Surgical Treatment of Atrial Fibrillation** 149
              Claudia M. Loardi, Marco Zanobini and Francesco Alamanni

              Permissions

              List of Contributors

              Index

Preface

The purpose of the book is to provide a glimpse into the dynamics and to present opinions and studies of some of the scientists engaged in the development of new ideas in the field from very different standpoints. This book will prove useful to students and researchers owing to its high content quality.

Cardiac arrhythmia is a group of conditions characterized by irregular, slow or fast heartbeat. It can be of four principal types- supraventricular tachycardias, bradyarrhythmias, ventricular arrhythmias and extra beats. Often, there are no noticeable symptoms in these diseases. However in serious cases, shortness of breath, chest pain, lightheadedness and passing out can occur. In other cases, cardiac arrest, stroke and heart failure may occur. An electrocardiogram and Holter monitor can prove to be definitive tests for cardiac arrhythmia. These conditions can be effectively treated with medications, medical procedures and surgery. Medications such as beta blockers and agents, and interventions such as the insertion of pacemakers and surgery may be used to restore normal heart rhythm. For severe symptoms of arrhythmia, cardioversion or defibrillation may be performed. This book contains some path-breaking studies revolving around cardiac arrhythmia. It unravels the recent studies in the mechanism pathways and management strategies of cardiac arrhythmia. For all readers who are interested in such studies, the case studies included in this book will serve as an excellent guide to develop a comprehensive understanding.

At the end, I would like to appreciate all the efforts made by the authors in completing their chapters professionally. I express my deepest gratitude to all of them for contributing to this book by sharing their valuable works. A special thanks to my family and friends for their constant support in this journey.

Editor

1

Breijo Electrocardiographic Pattern

Francisco R. Breijo-Márquez

Abstract

Breijo's electrocardiographic model is becoming better known to cardiologists every day. The decrease in the PR interval, together with the decrease of the QTc interval in the same ECG tracing, is the main and only cardiac electrical feature on the same individual. It can often go unnoticed, but many problems could be avoided if it was previously diagnosed, including sudden death.

Keywords: cardiac arrhythmias, Breijo pattern, sudden cardiac death, palpitations, tachycardia

1. Introduction

The decrease of the cardiac electrical systole—short PR and QTc intervals in the same electrocardiogram, also known as "Breijo electrocardiographic pattern"—is increasingly studied by several authors. The vast majority of the time it can be overlooked in an electrocardiogram tracing. More than 127 cases have been studied and cross-checked. Its diagnosis is essential in avoidance of the most heartbreaking consequence, that is, avoidable death. Despite the fact that for many authors, the cardiac electrical systole comprises only from the beginning of the Q wave to the end of the T wave, that is, depolarization and repolarization of the ventricles— the atria are also part of it. Therefore, the P wave, as well as the PR segment, must be a part of the electrical cardiac systole. When there is a shortening of the PR interval along with a shortening of the QT interval, we should talk about the *Decrease of cardiac electrical systole*. This peculiar electrocardiographic pattern is denominating the **Breijo pattern**: "A PR interval less than 0.120 s along with a QTc interval less than 0.360 s." It is typical in this type of patients, carriers of the **Breijo pattern**, to have some common peculiarities in all of them. 1. Unspecific symptoms that are considered mild, such as: Palpitations, usually nocturnal, which awaken the patient from the natural sleep. Profuse nocturnal sweating. Light-headedness feelings misinterpreted. 2. A feeling of chest pain very unspecified, not irradiated and whose electrocardiographic study is regarded, in the vast majority of cases, as nonspecific and atypical, since coronary alterations are not observed. 3. A personal background, in childhood, of seizures treated with antiepileptic drugs without the presence of an epileptic focus on the electroencephalogram. 4. Low levels of lythemia. 5. A preference for young age (up to 40) and male sex.

In 2008, Breijo-Marquez et al. [1–3] presented an electrocardiographic pattern, in which both the PR and QT intervals were shorter in milliseconds than what is regarded as acceptable limits.

They called this phenomenon as *Decrease of electrical cardiac systole"*[1], since both, depolarization and repolarization, atrial and ventricular, are lower in their standard lengths (PR interval and QT interval).

It is well known that, in an electrocardiogram, there are different waves, intervals, and segments.

They are as follows:

A. **Waves**: P, Q, R, S, T.

B. **Intervals**: PR (for other PQ authors). QRS. QT.

C. **Segments**: ST fundamentally.

In spite of the repeated repetition of the image, we put it below to gain a better understanding:

2. Normal electrocardiogram tracing

2.1. Waves: intervals and segments

The **P-wave** reflects atrial depolarization (contraction).

The **PR-interval** corresponds to the delay between the end of atrial depolarization (contraction) and the beginning of ventricular depolarization (contraction); its length must be between 0.120 s and 0.200 s.

The **Q wave** is a negative deflection in the ECG resulting at the beginning of ventricular depolarization (first wave in QRS complex).

The **T wave** is a reflection of ventricular repolarization.

The **QT interval** includes a complete ventricular depolarization and repolarization (full ventricular cycle); its length must be between 0.400 and 0.450 s (depending on authors and their conveniences since some authors have studied and published in different journals what the correct length of the QTc interval should be. Even they have not agreed with their different conclusions. We agree to Gollop, these values may vary; for us and with a broader context, the standard QTc values are between 0.400 and 0.450 s in length).

There are many formulas to measure the amount of these ranges; the most used are *Bazett and Fridericia* yet (**Figure 1**).

Like the R-R interval, the QT interval is dependent on the heart rate in an obvious way (the faster the heart rate, the shorter the R-R Interval and QT interval) and may be adjusted to improve the detection of patients at increased risk of ventricular arrhythmia.

The length of the PR (or PQ) interval, of the QRS complex, of the ST segment and the corrected QT interval, are all-important and must be valued in all cases.

The PR interval must be greater than 120 ms and lower than 200 ms.

Otherwise, we would find a **"short PR"** if this is fewer than 120 ms.

If greater than 200 ms, it would be denominated like an *Auricle-ventricular block in any of its variants.*

The QRS complex should have a maximum length of 0.10 s. If it were longer lasting, we would be in front of a branch block in its different modalities (complete or incomplete).

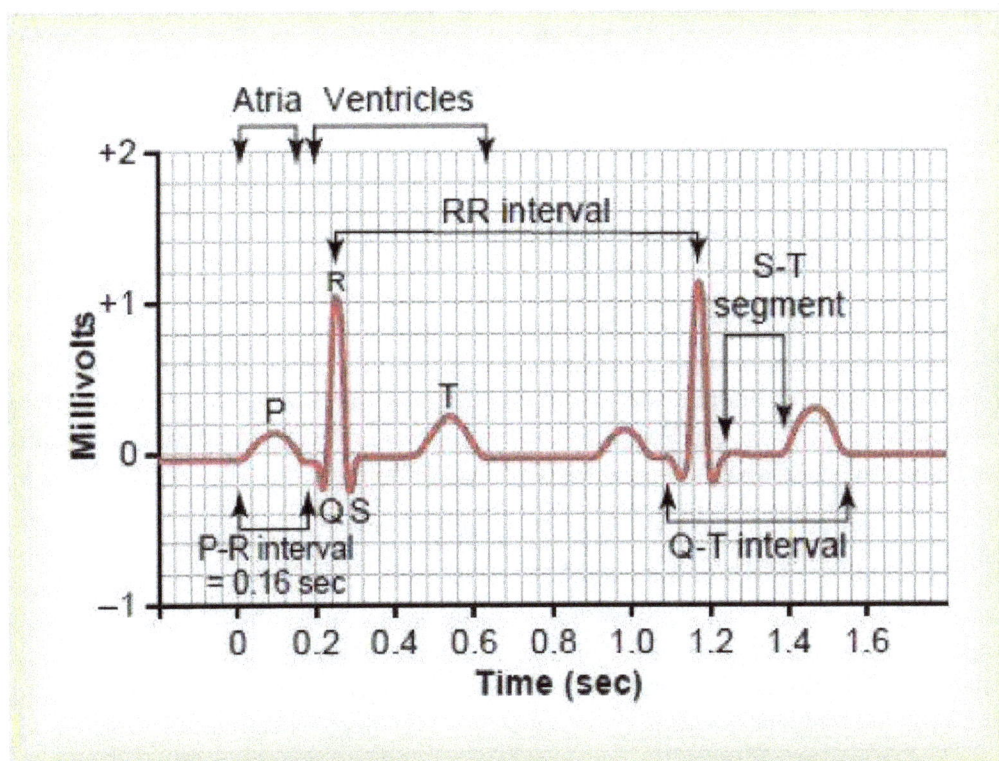

Figure 1. Graphical representation of a normal heart cycle. Indicating the waves, segments and intervals in time (abscissa) and millivolts (ordinate).

The great controversy that persists to this date is about which should be considered as an average length of the QT interval since it is related to the heart rate, that is, the QT value is frequency—dependent.

Several formulas are used to correct the QT interval (QTc). The most used are those of *Bazett and Fridericia.*

However, for these authors, typical values would be between 0.40 and 0.44 s, regardless of the person's age and sex.

The discrepancies among the different authors about the typical values of corrected QT are immense. These controversies are producing an authentic catastrophe when it comes to cataloging when it is or not a short QTC [4–8].

For us, in accordance with Gollop [9]—any QT value corrected interval less than 0.360 s must be considered as "short QT."

The most commonly used formulas are as follows (**Table 1**):

QT heart rate correction formulas	
Exponential	**Formula**
Bazett	QT/ RR1/2
Fridericia	QT/ RR1/3
Linear	**Formula**
Framingham	QT + 0.154 (1-RR)
Hodges	QT + 1.75 (HR-60)

Table 1. Formulas for QTc measure.

3. QT heart rate correction formulas

When the lengths of the different waves, intervals, and segments are greater or lesser than the values considered normal, the heart is much more vulnerable to arrhythmias. Any of these may be truly lethal, and accesses to ventricular fibrillation may develop.

As we have already mentioned, Breijo et al. published a new electrocardiographic pattern consisting of a short PR and QT intervals in the same electrocardiogram tracing.

People who had this kind of electrocardiographic pattern had also suffered from a wide variety of symptoms. Nocturnal tachycardias, dizziness, seizures, and unexplained syncopal accesses were the main symptoms common to all patients. They were diagnosed as people with epilepsy and treated with specific drugs for epilepsy; the results of such treatment were null.

However, the electroencephalographic registers did not provide any visualization for epileptic focus in any of the assessed patients. The patient age ranged from 16 to 40 years. The male gender was predominant. All previous electrocardiographic studies were considered within normal ranges.

As we have previously mentioned, the typical features of the **Breijo pattern** are:

1. A PR interval of fewer than 120 ms (short PR).

2. A QTc interval fewer than 360 ms.

Both on the same electrocardiographic tracing.

As we have mentioned previously, we agree with Gollop et al. [9] on when the QTc interval duration ought to be considered as "**short**."

Gollop et al. have written over 61 cases of Short QT Syndrome. Their cohort of 61 cases was predominantly male (75.4%) and had a mean QTc value of 0.306 s with values ranging from 0.248 to 0.381 s in symptomatic cases. For Gollop et al., the overall median age at clinical presentation was 21 years (adulthood) [IQR: 17–31.8 years) with a value of 20 years (IQR: 17–29 years) in males and 30 years (IQR: 19–44 years) in females].

These authors developed the ECG characteristics of the general population, and in consideration of clinical presentation, family history and genetic findings, a highly sensitive diagnostic using a scoring system.

This "scoring system" includes:

QTc in ms	
<370	1
<350	2
<330	3
J point-T peak interval	
<120	1
Clinical history	
Sudden cardiac arrest	2
Polymorphic VT or VF	2
Unexplained syncope	1
Atrial fibrillation	1
Family history	
First or second degree relative to SQTS	2
First or second degree relative to sudden death	1
Sudden infant death syndrome	1
Genotype	
Genotype positive	2
Mutation of undetermined significance in a culprit gene	1

Patients are deemed high probability (≥ 4 points), intermediate probability (3 points) or low probability (≤ 2 points).

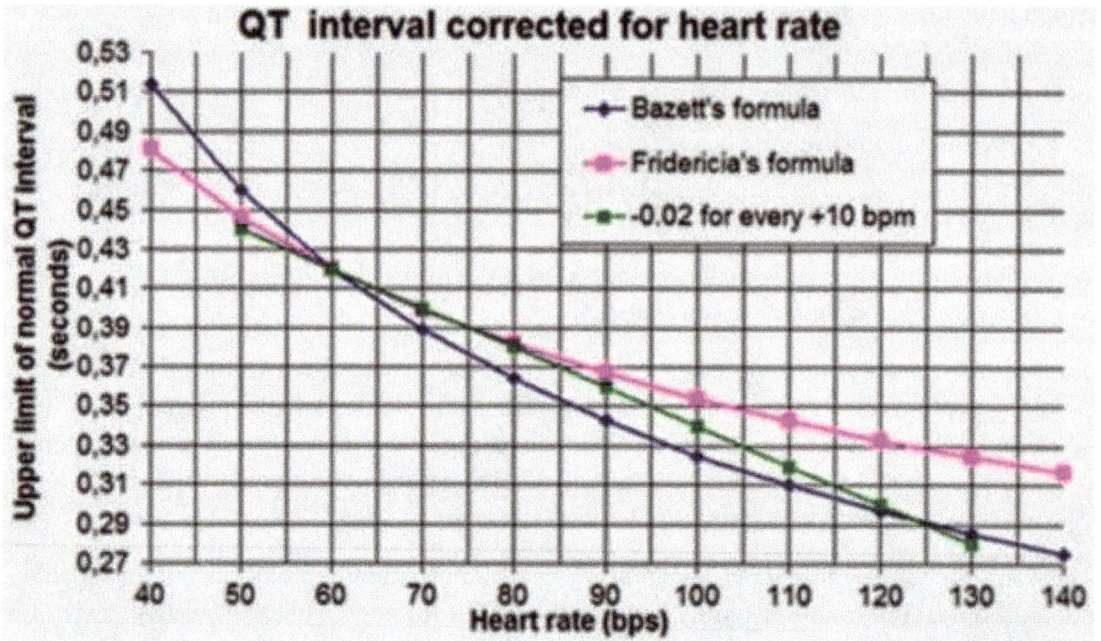

Figure 2. Boston Diagram.

Of all the current layouts, this is the one we consider as the most reliable and the most accurate.

We have seen cases of a short QT interval (QTc ≤ 0.350 s) in asymptomatic patients and without a positive family history thereto for congenital (and non-genetic) character.

We also think it is worthy to mention an interesting paradoxical ECG phenomenon called deceleration-dependent shortening of QT interval (shortening of QT interval associated with a decrease in heart rate); this should also be considered in a differential diagnosis [1–3].

In order to know precisely if the corrected QT value—by the different existing formulas—is in ranges, we use the **Boston diagram (Figure 2)**.

4. The Breijo pattern

As we have mentioned earlier, the first case of **Breijo pattern** was published in the International Journal of Cardiology in 2008.

The patient was a 37-year-old male, born in Mexico, D.F.

Since his childhood, he had suffered from tonic–clonic seizures and was treated with antiepileptic drugs (concretely with valproic acid) but without any epileptogenic focus showing up on his electroencephalogram.

Since then, the patient referred multiple accesses of nocturnal palpitations, accompanied by intense sweating that wet the pajamas. Feelings of gait instability. He liked to play sports, but at the minimum effort, he felt severe palpitations that impeded him from continuing with it.

The patient was anxious about his heart and visited numerous specialists in the field. He underwent a lot of diagnostic tests, and all of them were considered normal. The doctors believed him to be a patient with intense anxiety and hypochondriasis.

In two occasions, the patient suffered two syncope events that were considered vase-vagal etiology.

A thorough compilation of patients with this kind of symptoms such as infantile convulsions non-responders to conventional treatments, bouts of nocturnal tachycardia with sudden character, and syncopal events related to the effort.

An exhaustive study of personal antecedents, as well as your current clinical situation, was performed.

An exhaustive measurement of intervals, segments, and electrocardiographic waves. Measurement technique: MioLaserTool®, Pixruler® & Cardiocaliper®.

By way of example, we will expose the following case: A 37-year-old man with much nocturnal tachycardia crisis (since childhood) and three syncopal events observed and related to physical stress. In his family background, two sudden deaths were found: father died at age 55 of sudden cardiac, and a brother died at 22 months by sudden infant death.

He was diagnosed in his Reference Hospital (where he was transferred by emergency services) with supraventricular tachycardia to 195–200 beats/min (**Figure 3**), with narrow QRS

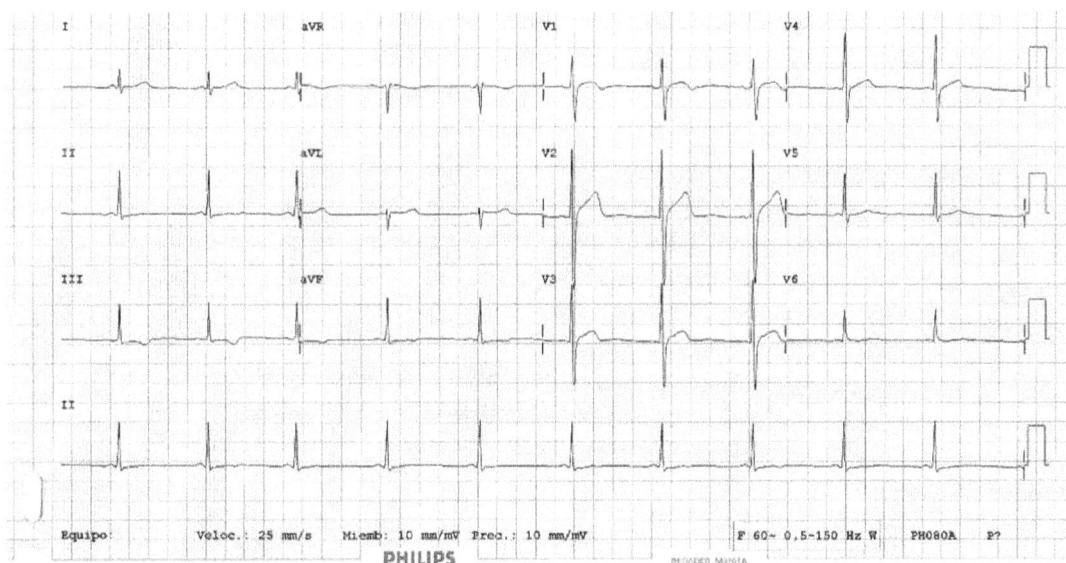

Figure 3. The full basal electrocardiogram tracing.

complexes. Severe diaphoresis, with the paleness of skin and mucous. A severe arterial hypotension to 90/50 mm Hg. Cardiac auscultation was in normal ranges but with a rapid rhythm. Tachypnea to 20 cycles/min. A grade Stuporous (Glasgow 15/15). The neurological examination was within normal ranges without focalizations. Central and peripheral pulses were palpable, symmetric, and synchronous in "frecuens". Supraventricular tachycardia disappeared using the administration of two doses of Adenosine i.v. in bolus, with six mgrs. Each one in 1 min (**Figure 4**). A hospital discharge was made after full stabilizing of acute process and patient was derived from your cardiologist outpatient, with the following diagnosis. A paroxysmal supraventricular tachycardia and Crisis of anxiety. The patient was transferred to our hospital because he had a similar event as the exposed, after the first visit with his outpatient cardiologist. There, the patient was adequately assessed with electrocardiogram, echocardiogram, blood levels of ions, and cardiac markers as well as electrophysiological study (EEF) (**Figure 5**). He was negative for high levels of Troponin (I-T), CK, CPK-MB; however, he was positive for low levels of lithium-ion (<0.1 mEq/L).

Nevertheless, in an in-depth and careful study of his basal electrocardiogram, we were able to assess the existence of a short PR and QTc interval.

Below, we present the first electrocardiogram of the patient that we were able to assess.

(Despite the fact that we practice a full series of tests on the patient, the most significant in this exposure is the electrocardiography and the Holter studies).

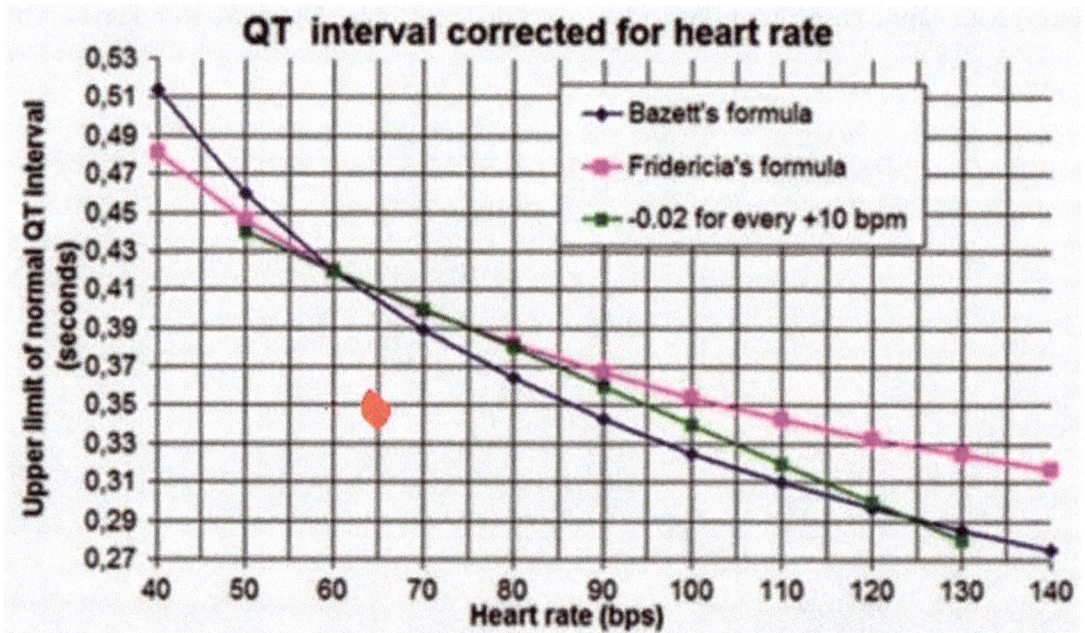

Figure 4. Graphic representation of the value obtained on the Boston diagram.

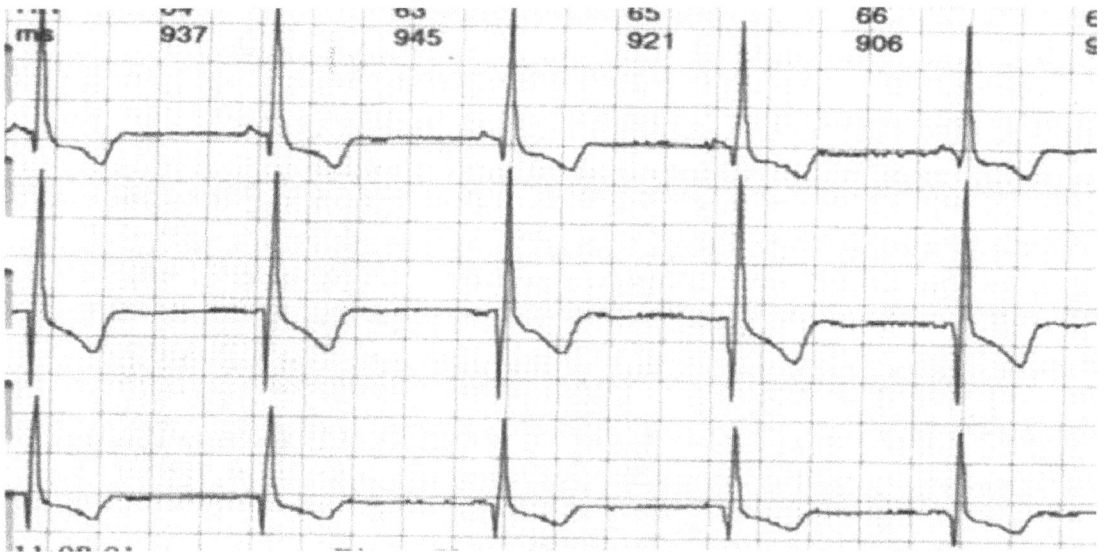

Figure 5. Same features as in Figure 1. PQ-interval: 0.100–0.110 s = Short PQ-interval. QTc (Bazzet) 0.339–0.340 s (< 0.350 s) = Short QT-interval. QTc (Fridericia) 0.332 s (< 0.350 s) = Short QT-interval.

In 60 bpm can be seen the short PR-interval (< 0.120 s) together in the short QT-interval (< 0.350 s.). Chiefly in inferior and precordial leads.

On the Boston Diagram, it would be (red marked).

5. Differential diagnosis

A differential diagnosis is imperative for any electrocardiographic entity that has a shortened PR interval.

These are fundamentally.

1. Wolff-Parkinson-White **(W P W)**.

2. Lown-Ganong-Levine **(LGL)**.

3. Mahaim.

Entity	PR-interval	QRS complex	QTc-interval
WPW	Short	Wide (δ-wave)	Normal
L.G.L	Short	Normal	Normal
Breijo pattern	Short	Normal	Short
Mahaim	Normal or short	Normal or wide	Normal

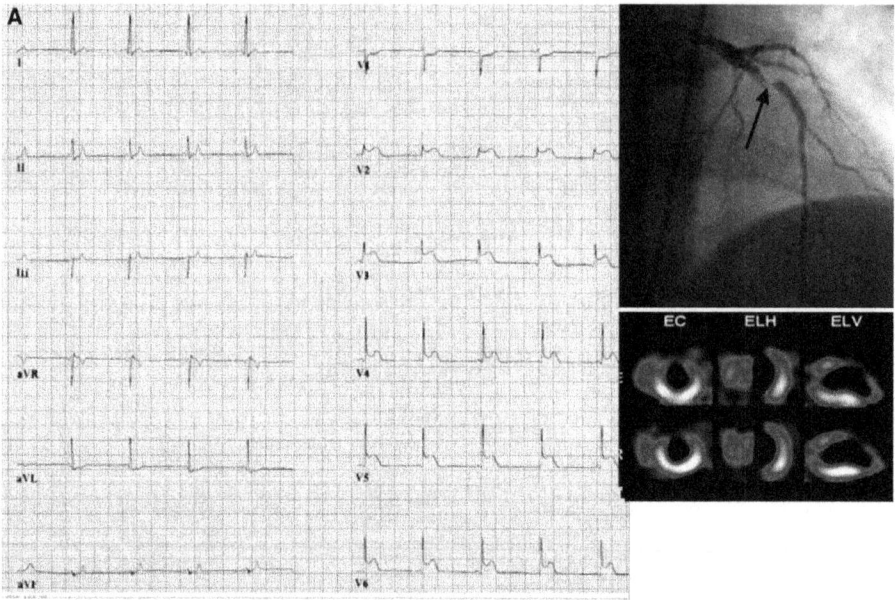

Figure 6. A **Breijo pattern** along with a *Wellens Pattern* can be valued in the image [10, 11].

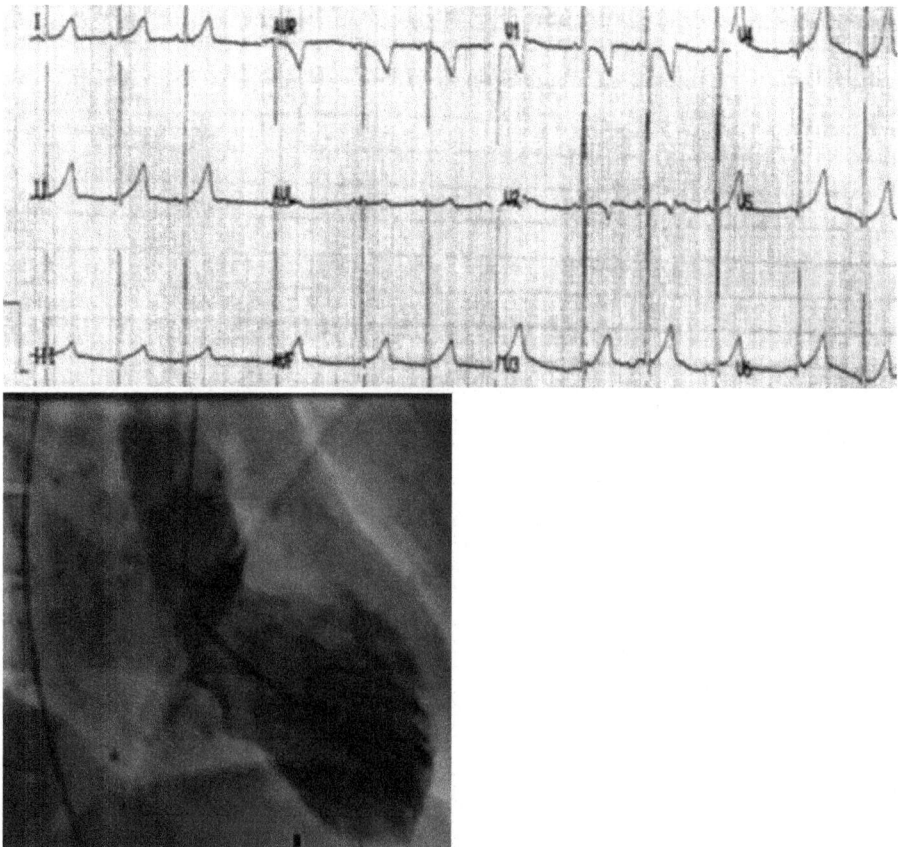

Figure 7. Electrocardiographic and arteriographic imaging of Takotsubo syndrome.

Differential diagnosis, based on the characteristics of the different intervals and complex.

This **"Breijo pattern"** we have assessed both in isolation and in association with other kinds of cardiac pathologies such as *"Wellens Pattern"*, *Wolf-Parkinson-White* syndrome and in *"Takotsubo's Disease"* as can be seen in **Figure 6**.

The *"Broken heart syndrome"* (**Takotsubo**) and the **Breijo pattern** are correctly appreciated in **Figure 7** [12, 13].

We have also known the existence of a *Wolf-Parkinson-White syndrome* associated with an electrocardiographic **Breijo pattern,** as can be seen in **Figure 8**.

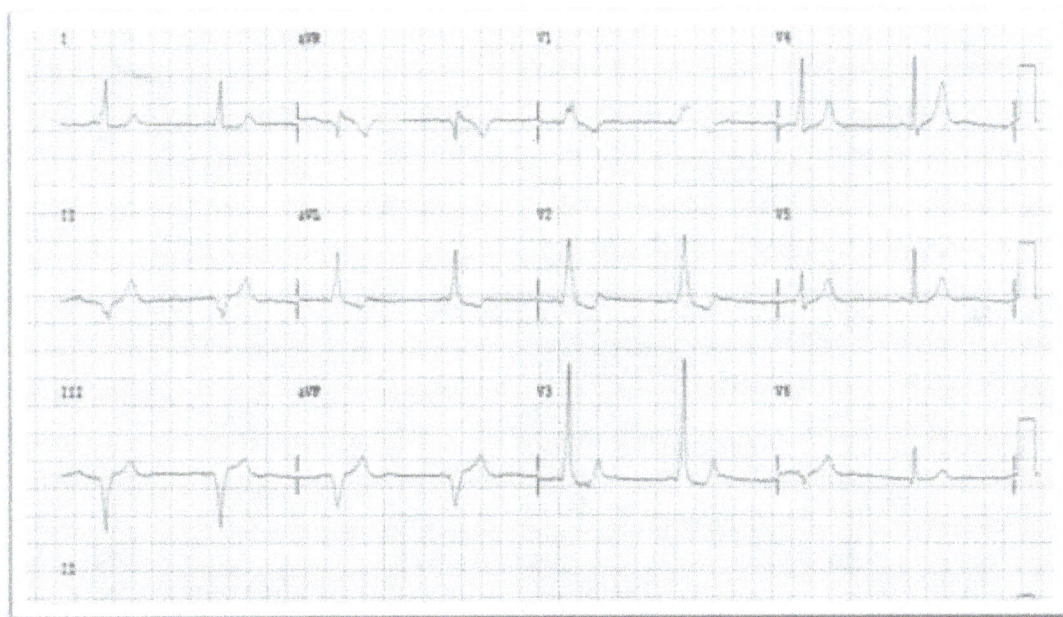

Figure 8. A *WPW* alongside a **Breijo pattern** can be perfectly seen in the image [14, 15].

RR	0.882352941176	seg
QTc (Rautaharju)	390	mseg
QTc (Bazett)	347	mseg
QTc (Framingham)	326	mseg
QTc (Friderica)	339	mseg
QTC (Call)	342	mseg

Table 2. Assessment of the values obtained according to the different formulas used.

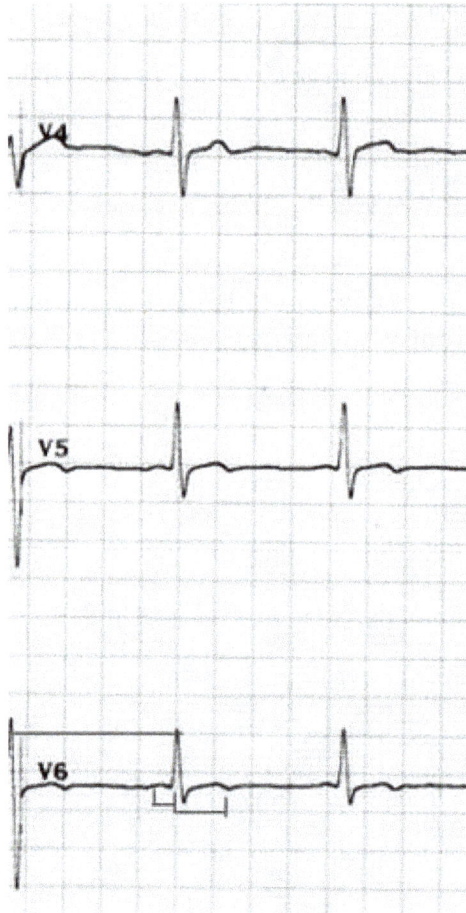

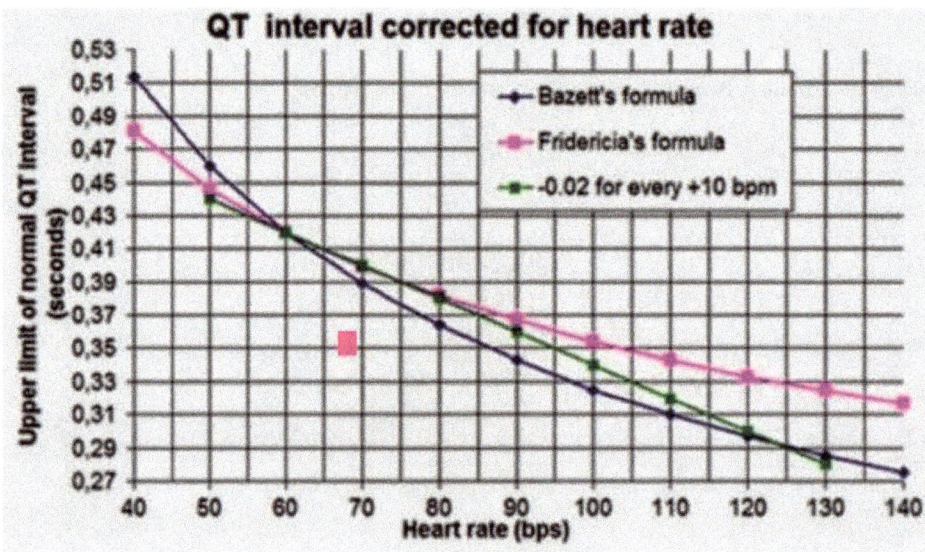

QT interval corrected for heart rate

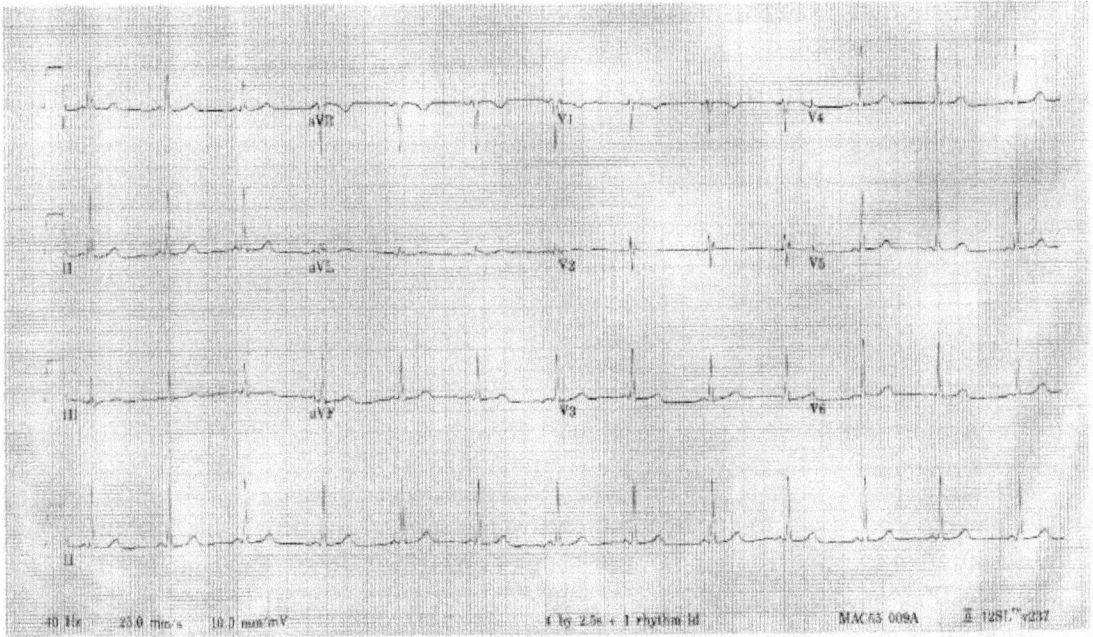

Figure 9. A full electrocardiogram performed with a Breijo pattern, in a male person.

6. Some significant images typical of the Breijo pattern

A typical image of a Breijo pattern in precordial left leads (**Table 2**).

Measured PR interval: 0.988 s.

Calculated QTc interval:

In the Boston diagram at 68 bpm.

** Square in red.

The last electrocardiogram performed with a **Breijo pattern**, in a male person who unfortunately died due to not being able to be recovered from a sudden death.

The electrocardiographic tracing was considered as within acceptable limits and his doctors decided to send him home (**Figure 9**).

PR interval value: 0.89 s (Very short).

Measured QTc value: Between 0.356 and 0.334 s very short).

In a nutshell, we can say the following about Breijo pattern as conclusions:

1. Although relatively little known so far, it is increasingly being discovered in ECG tracings that at first glance may appear normal.

2. The accurate reading of the ECG tracing must be of mandatory compliance. Despite the fact that symptoms referred by patients may be slight.

3. It is usually characteristic fact that most of the patients with a Breijo pattern have suffered in their childhood from seizure crisis without any focus of epilepsy being observed in all the assessed electroencephalography studies.

4. The most harmful consequence of the **Breijo pattern** is the sudden cardiac death, which, although fortunately does not occur often, can happen.

Summarizing:

- It is imperative to always take into account each and every symptom that a patient refers to, however slight they may seem to us. Especially if they are repetitive.

- Any patient who comes to our hospital with symptoms of nocturnal palpitations (which causes him/her to wake up from normal sleep), especially if they are accompanied by profuse sweating, nausea or throwing up, atypical thoracic discomfort as well as symptoms considered as mild or psychosomatic, especially if they are repetitive, should be evaluated in depth, without leaving any diagnostic elements ignored.

- Any patient with such characteristics must have a thorough examination of his or her background. Especially focused on the existence of syncopes or lost consciousness, as if the patient has suffered from convulsions in childhood, treated with antiepileptics and without focus electroencephalographic epileptogenic that can justify it.

- Carrying out an electrocardiographic study is imperative.

Assessing each and every one of its parameters. Making special emphasis on the lengths of the waves, intervals, and segments.

- The presence of a Breijo electrocardiographic pattern makes the heart much more vulnerable to severe arrhythmias and even sudden cardiac death.

- Whenever we find ourselves on an electrocardiogram with a short PR and QTc interval, we must be very alert and careful with the patient.

- Lithium levels in blood must be obligatorily assessed, since all patients with Pattern Breijo have low or very low levels.

Author details

Francisco R. Breijo-Márquez

Address all correspondence to: frbreijo@gmail.com

Clinical and Experimental Cardiology (on voluntary leave), East Boston Hospital Faculty of Medicine, Boston, MA, USA

References

[1] Breijo-Marquez FR. Decrease of electrical cardiac systole. International Journal of Cardiology. 2008;**126**(2, 23):e36-e38

[2] Breijo Marquez FR, Rios MP. Shortening of electrical cardiac systole: A new electrical disturbance? Short PR and QT intervals in the same electrocardiogram tracing (Breijo pattern). Journal of Cardiology and Current Research. 2014;**1**(1):00002

[3] Breijo-Marquez FR. Accelerated atrioventricular stimulation with an early and shortened ventricular repolarization in the same individual. WebmedCentral. Cardiology. 2014;**5**(3):WMC004589

[4] Zabel M, Franz MR, Klingenheben T, et al. Rate-dependence of QT dispersion and the QT interval: Comparison of atrial pacing and exercise testing. Journal of the American College of Cardiology. 2000;**36**:1654-1658

[5] Glancy JM, Garratt CJ, Woods KL, et al. Three-lead measurement of QTc dispersion. Journal of Cardiovascular Electrophysiology. 1995;**6**:987-992

[6] Behrens S, Li C, Knollmann BC, et al. Dispersion of ventricular repolarization in the voltage domain. Pacing and Clinical Electrophysiology. 1998;**21**:100-107

[7] Goldenberg I, Moss AJ, Wojciech Zareba MD. QT interval: How to measure it and what is "normal". Journal of Cardiovascular Electrophysiology. 2006;**17**(3):333-336

[8] Schwartz PJ, Moss AJ, Vincent GM, Crampton RS. Diagnostic criteria for the long QT syndrome. An update. Circulation. 1993;**88**(2):782-784

[9] Gollob MH, Redpath CJ, Roberts JD. The short QT syndrome: Proposed diagnostic criteria. Journal of the American College of Cardiology. 2011 Feb 15;**57**(7):802-812

[10] Tandy TK, Bottomy DP, Lewis JG. Wellens' syndrome. Annals of Emergency Medicine. 1999;**33**(3):347-351

[11] Breijo-Márquez FR, Ríos MP, Baños MA. Presence of a critical stenosis in left anterior descending coronary artery alongside a short "P-R" and "Q-T" pattern, in the same electrocardiographic record. Journal of Electrocardiology. 2010;**43**(5):422-424

[12] Vicenty A, Ortiz F, et al. Heart: Takotsubo cardiomyopathy. Boletín de la Asociación Médica de Puerto Rico. 2016;**108**(1):25-28

[13] Breijo-Marquez FR, Pardo Rios M. Sudden death in a patient with a short PR interval and subsequent sudden onset of a typical Tako-tsubo pattern. Open Journal of Internal Medicine. 2013;**3**:95-97

[14] Munger TM, Packer DL, Hammill SC, et al. A population study of the natural history of Wolff-Parkinson-White syndrome in Olmsted County, Minnesota, 1953-198. Circulation. 1993;**87**(3):866-873

[15] Breijo-Marquez FR. A Breijo pattern associated to a Wolff-Parkinson-White pattern. Journal of Cardiology and Current Research. 2016;**5**(3):00161

2

Histopathological Change Following Cox-Maze IV Procedure for Atrial Fibrillation

Takashi Murashita

Abstract

The prevalence of atrial fibrillation and the likelihood of undergoing concomitant surgical ablation at the time of open heart surgery are increasing. Currently, the conventional cut-and-sew Maze procedure has been predominantly replaced by Cox-Maze IV procedure, in which new energy sources such as radiofrequency energy and/or cryoablation are applied. Cox-Maze IV procedure has been associated with lower rate of complications than a cut-and-sew procedure. However, some previous studies reported the lower success rate of Cox-Maze IV procedure, possibly because radiofrequency ablation or cryoablation cannot always achieve transmurality. For the success of surgical ablation, achieving transmurality, defined as complete atrial wall thickness of fibrotic changes, is of paramount importance. A review of previous articles regarding histopathological changes of the atrial tissue following surgical ablation is performed. The effectiveness of new energy sources such as radiofrequency and cryoablation in terms of histological transmurality is discussed.

Keywords: atrial fibrillation, Maze procedure, radiofrequency, cryoablation

1. Introduction

Surgical ablation for atrial fibrillation (AF) has been under continuous development for over two decades. The most recent guidelines for the surgical treatment of AF reported by the Society of Thoracic Surgeons (STS) state that surgical ablation for persistent AF can be performed without adding operative risk and is recommended at the time of concomitant mitral valve operations, isolated aortic valve operations, isolated coronary artery bypass grafting, and combined aortic valve and coronary artery bypass surgery (class I strength of recommendation) [1]. Surgical ablation is also recommended to symptomatic AF refractory to medical or catheter-based therapy in the absence of structural heart disease (class II strength of recommendation) [1].

Cox Maze Procedure

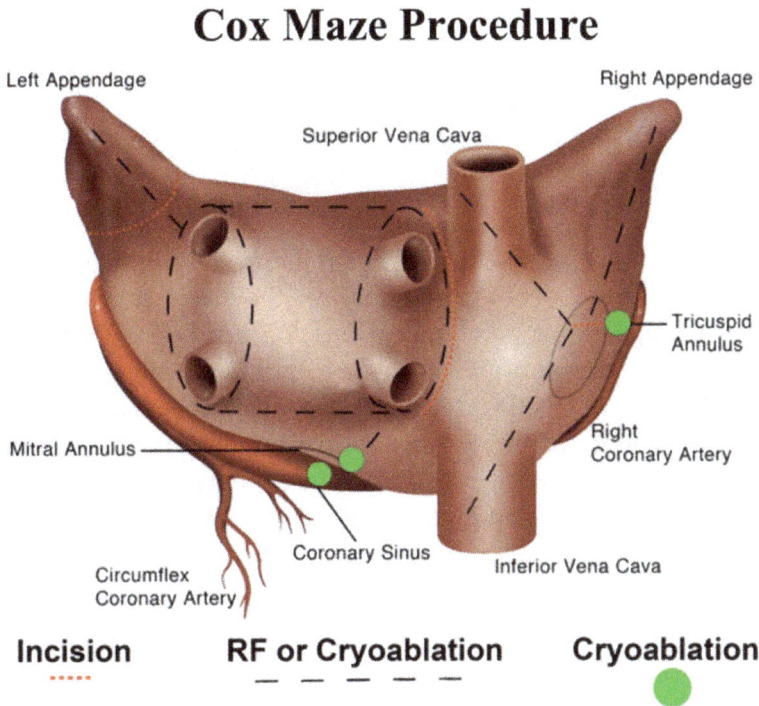

Figure 1. Scheme of the bi-atrial Cox-Maze procedure IV utilizing radiofrequency (RF) or cryoablation energy sources.

The first clinical surgical ablation for AF was introduced by Dr. James Cox in 1987, and was termed the Cox-Maze I. The successful 22 cases were reported in 1991 [2]. Over the subsequent years, the operation evolved into the Cox-Maze III or the cut-and-sew Maze [3], which has been applied extensively in clinical practice [4]. In the meantime, the introduction of ablation technology has significantly changed the attitude. Damiano et al. employed a combination of radiofrequency energy and cryoablation to replace several of the Cox-Maze III cut and sew lesions and termed this procedure as the Cox-Maze IV [5, 6]. Finally, the lesion sets of the Cox-Maze IV have evolved to its current form [7, 8] (**Figure 1**).

Khargi et al. reported that conventional cut-and-sew Cox-Maze III procedure is getting less frequently performed, and alternative sources of energy were predominantly used in all surgical ablation cases (92.0%), and almost always (98.4%) in concomitant procedures [9]. Cryoablation is employed as an alternative source of energy [10–12]. As compared to radiofrequency and cryoablation, other energy sources such as microwave, laser, and high-frequency ultrasound have proven less effective, and are not commercially available now [13–18].

2. Electrophysiologic basis of atrial fibrillation

It was documented that all AF is characterized by the presence of two or more large macroreentrant circuits in the atria simultaneously [19]. Haïssaguerre et al. first detected the focal triggers of atrial ectopic beats [20]. They noted that the ectopic foci are mainly (>90%) located in and around the orifices of the pulmonary veins and the remaining are located in other sites such as right atrium, left atrium, crista terminalis, and left atrial appendage. The findings of their paper, which reported that the triggers were successfully treated with radiofrequency ablation, led to an explosion of efforts by a number of cardiologists and cardiac surgeons to treat AF with catheter ablation and surgical techniques, respectively. The concept of treating AF was originally focused on isolating the pulmonary veins, either by catheters or surgical devices.

However, AF produces unfavourable changes in atrial function and structure, which is called remodeling [21]. After many years of paroxysmal AF, the macroreentrant circuits of AF can become self-perpetuating. At this point, paroxysmal AF can become long-standing or persistent AF, and the underlying electrophysiologic culprit is no longer the focal triggers, but rather the macroreentrant circuits themselves. Therefore, for long-standing or persistent AF, simple isolation of pulmonary veins is not an effective treatment because the focal triggers do not account for onset of AF for this type of AF. In these patients, it is necessary to interrupt the macroreentrant circuits by placing additional linear lesions in the atria. This concept has led to a surgical ablation technique called Cox-Maze procedure.

3. Cryoablation

3.1. Introduction of cryoablation

The era of cryosurgery began with the development of automated cryosurgical equipment in the 1960s. Cooper et al. described cryosurgical resection of parenchymal organs using liquid nitrogen-refrigerated clamp in 1966 [22]. Cryosurgery has been an integral part of the surgical treatment of cardiac arrhythmias since the 1970s. With the recent technological development of cryoablation devices, the use of cryothermy in the treatment of cardiac arrhythmias is increasing.

Cryoablation is effective in producing electrical silent ablation lines, and can be used judiciously safely without injuring surrounding structures such as coronary arteries and valve tissue.

3.2. Mechanisms of tissue injury in cryoablation

Gage et al. described the mechanisms of tissue injury in cryosurgery [23]. The adverse effect of low temperature on cells begins as temperature falls into the hypothermic range. The function and structure of cells are stressed, and cell metabolism progressively fails. As the temperature goes further down and falls into the freezing range, water is crystallized, which causes more serious consequences than the earlier cooling. Ice crystal formation first occurs in the extracellular spaces, and with further cooling, it occurs within the cell. Intracellular ice formation requires temperatures colder than −40°C. Once intracellular ice is formed, it disrupts organelles and cell membranes, and cell death is practically certain.

The progress to a stable lesion can be divided into three phases: (1) freeze/thaw phase, (2) haemorrhagic and inflammatory phase, and (3) replacement fibrosis phase [24].

1. Freeze/thaw phase.

   Intracellular and extracellular ice formation vary in size and location depending on tissue type, proximity to the cryoprobe, and the presence of blood flow during cryoablation. Ice crystals, themselves, do not cause mechanical disruption. They do not penetrate the cell membrane, but induce compression and distortion of adjacent cytoplasmic components [25, 26]. Irreversible injury to mitochondria is a consequence of increased membrane permeability during the thaw phase [27]. The damage to the mitochondrial membrane leads to membrane lipid peroxidation and enzyme hydrolysis. At this point, mitochondria become irreversibly deenergized [28]. In the heart, the application of cryoprobe to myocardium results in the formation of an elliptical hemispheroid lesion [29]. During the thawing, the myocytes get swollen and the myofilaments are extremely stretched.

2. Haemorrhagic and inflammatory phase.

   The second phase of myocardial injury following cryoablation is characterized by the development of haemorrhage [29], oedema, and inflammation [30], which are found within 48 hours after thawing. Harrison et al. reported the histologic changes following cryoablation to the atrioventricular node [31]. One week after the procedure, microscopy showed necrosis of myocardial cells and conduction fibres, a polymorphonuclear leukocytic infiltrate and marked haemorrhage in the peripheral lesion.

3. Replacement fibrosis phase.

   The last phase in the evolution of a stable cryolesion is detected at 2–4 weeks after the cryoablation. At this point, the cryolesions consist of dense collagen and fat infiltration along with many small blood vessels. Harrison et al. reported that, 1 month after the procedure, the lesion had been replaced by dense fibrotic connective tissue [31].

3.3. Electrophysiologic effects of cryoablation on the heart

Jensen et al. developed an experimental myocardial injury model using cryoinjury in dogs [32]. Their histologic examination showed that the cellular pattern or healing myocardial cryolesions was similar to that of a healing myocardial infarction, but with less variability. Several papers reported that cryolesions have low arrhythmogenic potential in canine models [33–35].

Holman et al. reported the decrease of electrogram amplitude in cryolesions [33]. The decrease in amplitude reflects epicardial ice insulation or inhibition of myocardial electrical potential. More than 70% decrease in absolute amplitude from control potentials was predictive of cellular death. Klein et al. demonstrated that the cryolesions are sharply demarcated from normal myocardium and does not disrupt the surrounding anatomy [34]. The chronic cryolesion behaves electrophysiologically like an inert plug with no disruption of surrounding activation. Ventricular ectopic activity disappeared in cryolesions after 1 week of the cryoablation.

In conclusion, the cryothermal energy can create discrete, structurally intact, and electrically inert foci in the myocardium. That is, the electrophysiologic mechanism for a cryoablation is considered to be a useful therapeutic modality in the treatment of cardiac arrhythmias.

3.4. Cryoablation device

Cryothermal energy is delivered to myocardial tissue by using a cryoprobe. Cryoablation devices create an inflammatory response (cryonecrosis) that blocks the electrical conduction pathway by freezing target tissues.

There are two commercially available cryoablation probes for surgical treatment of cardiac arrhythmias. AtriCure Inc. (Mason, OH) has provided cryoICE probe, which uses a 10 cm malleable probe on a 20 cm shaft. It utilizes nitrous oxide (N_2O) to create continuous transmural lesions that block propagation of atrial activation. The cryoFORM is a latest generation of cryoablation probe, which is made from stainless steel and has a corrugated surface, a design that provides a high flexibility [36] (**Figure 2**).

Medtonic Inc. (Minneapolis, MN) has developed Cardioblate CryoFlex surgical ablation probes, which utilize argon-powered cryoablation (**Figure 3**). This is a malleable probe easily shaped by hand, and reaches temperature of approximately −150°C. This device is currently approved for use in surgical ablation for AF in Europe but not in the United States.

3.5. Transmurality of cryoablation

Kettering et al. created a successful, a right atrial septal linear lesion with cryocatheter in pigs [37]. The bipolar voltage map demonstrated very low potentials along the ablation line and a sharply demarcated ablation area. However, they concluded that creating a transmural lesion and a complete conduction block remains an unsolved problem. Wadhwa et al. reported that successful transmurality was achieved with catheter cryoablation in the canine ventricle [38]. Masroor et al. reported that endocardial hypothermia was achieved with epicardial

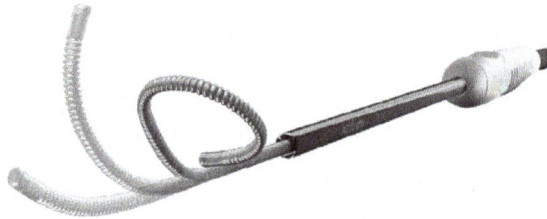

Figure 2. Illustration of the flexibility of the cryoFORM ablation probe. The length of the active site of the malleable probe surface is adjustable by the movable shaft cover (Reproduced with permission from AtriCure, Inc.).

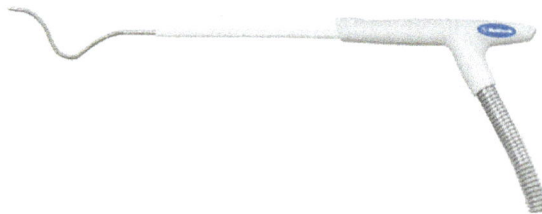

Figure 3. Illustration of the Cardioblate CryoFlex ablation device (Reproduced with permission from Medtronic, Inc.).

cryoablation on a beating heart model in pigs [39]. Schill et al. reported that the latest cryoablation probe produced transmural lesions in 97% of the arrested heart in an ovine model [40].

However, the transmurality created by surgical cryoablation in the human tissue has not been well studied.

4. Radiofrequency ablation

4.1. Introduction of radiofrequency ablation

Since Haissaguerre et al. demonstrated the efficacy of radiofrequency ablation for paroxysmal atrial fibrillation [20], radiofrequency has become the standard treatment for both catheter-based ablation and surgical ablation for cardiac arrhythmias. Chiappini et al. reported the efficacy of radiofrequency ablation in the patients who had chronic atrial fibrillation, and it was as effective as cut-and-sew Maze procedure [41, 42].

However, lesions created by hyperthermia have a potential risk of tissue disruption that can result in perforation of surrounding tissue, pulmonary stenosis, and thromboembolic stroke [43, 44].

4.2. Bipolar versus unipolar radiofrequency

Bugge et al. compared the transmurality of ablated lesions in ovine hearts using irrigated bipolar and unipolar radiofrequency ablation [45]. They reported that bipolar radiofrequency was superior in creating transmurality, but both devices failed to produce consistent transmurality using the epicardial beating heart technique. Gonzalez-Suarez et al. also demonstrated that bipolar is more effective than unipolar in achieving transmurality in vitro [46]. However, the superiority of bipolar over unipolar in human has not been established.

AtriCure Inc. (Mason, OH) has provided bipolar radiofrequency ablation device, which has stainless steel shaft and jaws to maintain consistent tissue pressure and precise electrode alignment across the entire length of the jaws (**Figure 4**).

Medtonic Inc. (Minneapolis, MN) has provided Cardioblate system, which utilizes irrigated bipolar radiofrequency energy to ablate tissue transmurally (**Figure 5**).

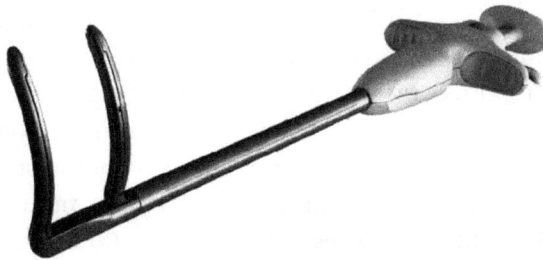

Figure 4. Illustration of the bipolar radiofrequency clamp (Reproduced with permission from AtriCure, Inc.).

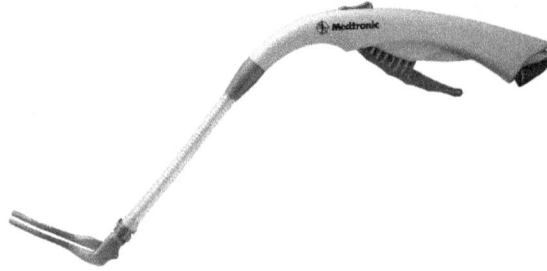

Figure 5. Illustration of the Cardioblate clamp, which utilizes bipolar radiofrequency energy source (Reproduced with permission from Medtronic, Inc.).

4.3. Histopathological changes after radiofrequency ablation

Heat propagation is based on both resistive and passive mechanisms. In the early phase of radiofrequency ablation, tissue is heated to 50–60°C resulting in coagulation and irreversible destruction of cell and collagen structures. Ablation of the peripheral part of the lesion results from passive heating with the same effect of irreversible damage. Both resistive and passive heating propagate in all directions so that the tissue lesion becomes similar in depth and width [41]. Once the transmurality is achieved with radiofrequency ablation, there is no proarrhythmic activity found in the scar tissue [47].

Aupperle et al. reported the histological findings in experimental atrial ablation in sheep [48]. They reported that epicardial bipolar radiofrequency resulted in intensive endocardial necroses and severe sharply demarcated transmural myocardial necroses. Similarly, endocardial unipolar radiofrequency resulted in severe endocardial necroses as well as intense, transmural, and well demarcated myocardial necroses. Ba et al. also reported that radiofrequency resulted in myocyte necrosis in sheep, and radiofrequency was as effective as cryotherapy [49]. Gaynor et al. performed surgical ablation using bipolar radiofrequency energy source in pigs [50]. They reported histological assessment that showed all lesions created by bipolar radiofrequency were transmural and there were no stenosis of the coronary vessels or injuries to the valves.

4.4. Transmurality of radiofrequency ablation

Although bipolar radiofrequency produces transmural linear lesions in the animals [51, 52], transmurality is not always achieved in human, as several papers reported [53, 54]. Deneke et al. reported that transmurality of the ablated lesions could only be found in 75% in human atria [55]. Kasirajan et al. reported the histopathological findings in three human patients who had autopsy after surgical ablation [53]. Their microscopic examination showed that (1) surgically ablated lesions showed not only transmural but also nontransmural lesions (**Figure 6**), (2) chronic ischemic and fibrotic changes existed in the myocardium of the patients who had long-standing persistent AF and mitral regurgitation, and (3) acute bi-directional electrical conduction block did not guarantee transmurality of ablation lesions. They assumed that the underlying disease process prevented the creation of transmural lesions. The wall thickness

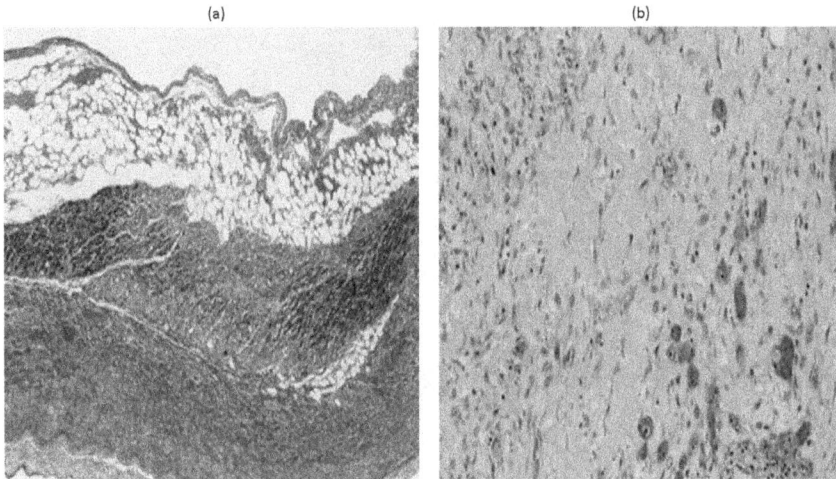

Figure 6. (a) Day 6 of surgical ablation. Extensive fibrosis in atrial tissue (blue) with necrotic myocardium (purple), and viable muscle (red). (Mason trichrome stain: magnification ×40.) (b) Day 18 of surgical ablation. Healing with coagulative necrosis and wavy bundles of collagen with few viable cells in between (hematoxylin and eosin: magnification ×100.).

of the atrium has been known to affect the transmurality [45]. Therefore, repeated radiofrequency ablation is recommended, especially in thick lesions [56, 57].

Ventosa-Fernandez et al. reported the histologic evidence of transmurality 4 years after bipolar radiofrequency ablation [58].

5. Conclusions

Recently, the conventional cut-and-sew Cox-Maze procedure has been replaced by alternative energy sources in the surgical treatment of atrial fibrillation. Cryoablation and radiofrequency ablation have been playing an important role in this field. Both energy sources have been shown to be effective in treating atrial fibrillation. However, despite the technological advancement, there remains uncertainty of transmurality in human tissue, especially when patients have underlying disease. Lack of transmurality may result in failure of surgical ablation. Further histopathological studies will be necessary in assessing the effectiveness of using alternative energy sources. Moreover, a further technological advancement in achieving reliable transmurality should be warranted in the future.

Author details

Takashi Murashita

Address all correspondence to: tmurashita@gmail.com

West Virginia University, Heart and Vascular Institute, Morgantown, WV, USA

References

[1] Badhwar V, Rankin J, Damiano R Jr, Gillinov A, Bakaeen F, Edgerton J, Philpott J, McCarthy P, Bolling S, Roberts H, Thourani V, Suri R, Shemin R, Firestone S, Ad N. The Society of Thoracic Surgeons 2017 clinical practice guidelines for the surgical treatment of atrial fibrillation. The Annals of Thoracic Surgery. 2017;**103**:329-341. DOI: 10.1016/j. athoracsur.2016.10.076

[2] Cox J, Boineau J, Schuessler R, Ferguson T Jr, Cain M, Lindsay B, Corr P, Kater K, Lappas D. Successful surgical treatment of atrial fibrillation. Review and clinical update. Journal of the American Medical Association. 1991;**266**:1976-1980

[3] Cox J, Schuessler R, Lappas D, Boineau J. An 8 1/2-year clinical experience with surgery for atrial fibrillation. Annals of Surgery. 1996;**224**:267-273

[4] Millar R, Arcidi J Jr, Alison P. The maze III procedure for atrial fibrillation: Should the indications be expanded? The Annals of Thoracic Surgery. 2000;**70**:1580-1586

[5] Mokadam N, McCarthy P, Gillinov A, Ryan W, Moon M, Mack M, Gaynor S, Prasad S, Wickline S, Bailey M, Damiano N, Ishii Y, Schuessler R, Damiano R Jr. A prospective multicenter trial of bipolar radiofrequency ablation for atrial fibrillation: Early results. The Annals of Thoracic Surgery. 2004;**78**:1665-1670. DOI: 10.1016/j.athoracsur.2004.05.066

[6] Gaynor S, Diodato M, Prasad S, Ishii Y, Schuessler R, Bailey M, Damiano N, Bloch J, Moon M, Damiano R Jr. A prospective, single-center clinical trial of a modified Cox maze procedure with bipolar radiofrequency ablation. The Journal of Thoracic and Cardiovascular Surgery. 2004;**128**:535-542. DOI: 10.1016/j.jtcvs.2004.02.044

[7] Damiano R Jr, Schwartz F, Bailey M, Maniar H, Munfakh N, Moon M, Schuessler R. The Cox maze IV procedure: Predictors of late recurrence. The Journal of Thoracic and Cardiovascular Surgery. 2011;**141**:113-121. DOI: 10.1016/j.jtcvs.2010.08.067

[8] Cheema F, Younus M, Pasha A, Cox J, Roberts H Jr. An effective modification to simplify the right atrial lesion set of the Cox-cryomaze. The Annals of Thoracic Surgery. 2013;**96**:330-332. DOI: 10.1016/j.athoracsur.2012.12.065

[9] Khargi K, Hutten B, Lemke B, Deneke T. Surgical treatment of atrial fibrillation; a systematic review. European Journal of Cardio-Thoracic Surgery. 2005;**27**:258-265. DOI: 10.1016/j.ejcts.2004.11.003

[10] Ad N, Henry L, Hunt S. The concomitant cryosurgical Cox-maze procedure using Argon based cryoprobes: 12 month results. The Journal of Cardiovascular Surgery. 2011;**52**:593-599

[11] Gammie J, Laschinger J, Brown J, Poston R, Pierson R 3rd, Romar L, Schwartz K, Santos M, Griffith BA. Multi-institutional experience with the CryoMaze procedure. The Annals of Thoracic Surgery. 2005;**80**:876-880. DOI: 10.1016/j.athoracsur.2005.03.075

[12] Gaita F, Riccardi R, Caponi D, Shah D, Garberoglio L, Vivalda L, Dulio A, Chiecchio A, Manasse E, Gallotti R. Linear cryoablation of the left atrium versus pulmonary vein

cryoisolation in patients with permanent atrial fibrillation and valvular heart disease: Correlation of electroanatomic mapping and long-term clinical results. Circulation. 2005;**111**:136-142. DOI: 10.1161/01.CIR.0000151310.00337.FA

[13] Molloy T. Midterm clinical experience with microwave surgical ablation of atrial fibrillation. The Annals of Thoracic Surgery. 2005;**79**:2115-2118. DOI: 10.1016/j.athoracsur.2004.06.104

[14] Pruitt J, Lazzara R, Ebra G. Minimally invasive surgical ablation of atrial fibrillation: The thoracoscopic box lesion approach. Journal of Interventional Cardiac Electrophysiology. 2007;**20**:83-87. DOI: 10.1007/s10840-007-9172-3

[15] Lin Z, Shan Z, Liao C, Chen L. The effect of microwave and bipolar radio-frequency ablation in the surgical treatment of permanent atrial fibrillation during valve surgery. The Thoracic and Cardiovascular Surgeon. 2011;**59**:460-464. DOI: 10.1055/s-0030-1271146

[16] MacDonald D, Maruthappu M, Nagendran M. How effective is microwave ablation for atrial fibrillation during concomitant cardiac surgery? Interactive Cardiovascular and Thoracic Surgery. 2012;**15**:122-127. DOI: 10.1093/icvts/ivs137

[17] Klinkenberg T, Ahmed S, Ten Hagen A, Wiesfeld A, Tan E, Zijlstra F, Van Gelder I. Feasibility and outcome of epicardial pulmonary vein isolation for lone atrial fibrillation using minimal invasive surgery and high intensity focused ultrasound. Europace. 2009;**11**:1624-1631. DOI: 10.1093/europace/eup299

[18] Basu S, Nagendran M, Maruthappu M. How effective is bipolar radiofrequency ablation for atrial fibrillation during concomitant cardiac surgery? Interactive Cardiovascular and Thoracic Surgery. 2012;**15**:741-748. DOI: 10.1093/icvts/ivs311

[19] Cox J. A brief overview of surgery for atrial fibrillation. Annals of Cardiothoracic Surgery. 2014;**3**:80-88. DOI: 10.3978/j.issn.2225-319X.2014.01.05

[20] Haïssaguerre M, Jaïs P, Shah D, Takahashi A, Hocini M, Quiniou G, Garrigue S, Le Mouroux A, Le Métayer P, Clémenty J. Spontaneous initiation of atrial fibrillation by ectopic beats originating in the pulmonary veins. The New England Journal of Medicine. 1998;**339**:659-666. DOI: 10.1056/NEJM199809033391003

[21] Allessie M, Ausma J, Schotten U. Electrical, contractile and structural remodeling during atrial fibrillation. Cardiovascular Research. 2002;**54**:230-246

[22] Cooper I, Hirose T. Application of cryogenic surgery to resection of parenchymal organs. The New England Journal of Medicine. 1966;**274**:15-18. DOI: 10.1056/NEJM196601062740103

[23] Gage A, Baust J. Mechanisms of tissue injury in cryosurgery. Cryobiology. 1998;**37**:171-186. DOI: 10.1006/cryo.1998.2115

[24] Lustgarten D, Keane D, Ruskin J. Cryothermal ablation: Mechanism of tissue injury and current experience in the treatment of tachyarrhythmias. Progress in Cardiovascular Diseases. 1999;**41**:481-498

[25] Gill W, Fraser J, Carter D. Repeated freeze-thaw cycles in cryosurgery. Nature. 1968;**219**:410-413

[26] Whittaker D. Mechanisms of tissue destruction following cryosurgery. Annals of the Royal College of Surgeons of England. 1984;**66**:313-318

[27] Tsvetkov T, Tsonev L, Meranzov N, Minkov I. Functional changes in mitochondrial properties as a result of their membrane cryodestruction. II. Influence of freezing and thawing on ATP complex activity of intact liver mitochondria. Cryobiology. 1985;**22**:111-118

[28] Petrenko A. A mechanism of latent cryoinjury and reparation of mitochondria. Cryobiology. 1992;**29**:144-152

[29] Holman W, Ikeshita M, Douglas J, Smith P, Cox J. Cardiac cryosurgery: Effects of myocardial temperature on cryolesion size. Surgery. 1983;**93**:268-272

[30] Mikat E, Hackel D, Harrison L, Gallagher J, Wallace A. Reaction of the myocardium and coronary arteries to cryosurgery. Laboratory Investigation. 1977;**37**:632-641

[31] Harrison L, Gallagher J, Kasell J, Anderson R, Mikat E, Hackel D, Wallace A. Cryosurgical ablation of the A-V node-His bundle: A new method for producing A-V block. Circulation. 1977;**55**:463-470

[32] Jensen J, Kosek J, Hunt T, Goodson W, Miller D. Cardiac cryolesions as an experimental model of myocardial wound healing. Annals of Surgery. 1987;**206**:798-803

[33] Holman W, Ikeshita M, Douglas J, Smith P, Lofland G, Cox J. Ventricular cryosurgery: Short-term effects on intramural electrophysiology. The Annals of Thoracic Surgery. 1983;**35**:386-393

[34] Klein G, Harrison L, Ideker R, Smith W, Kasell J, Wallace A, Gallagher J. Reaction of the myocardium to cryosurgery: Electrophysiology and arrhythmogenic potential. Circulation. 1979;**59**:364-372

[35] Hunt G, Chard R, Johnson D, Ross D. Comparison of early and late dimensions and arrhythmogenicity of cryolesions in the normothermic canine heart. The Journal of Thoracic and Cardiovascular Surgery. 1989;**97**:313-318

[36] Schroeter T, Misfeld M. Characteristics of the new AtriCure cryoFORM® cryoablation probe for the surgical treatment of cardiac arrhythmias. Expert Review of Medical Devices. 2017;**14**:255-262. DOI: 10.1080/17434440.2017.1309972

[37] Kettering K, Al-Ghobainy R, Wehrmann M, Vonthein R, Mewis C. Atrial linear lesions: Feasibility using cryoablation. Pacing and Clinical Electrophysiology. 2006;**29**:283-289. DOI: 10.1111/j.1540-8159.2006.00335.x

[38] Wadhwa M, Rahme M, Dobak J, Li H, Wolf P, Chen P, Feld G. Transcatheter cryoablation of ventricular myocardium in dogs. Journal of Interventional Cardiac Electrophysiology. 2000;**4**:537-545

[39] Masroor S, Jahnke M, Carlisle A, Cartier C, Lalonde J, Macneil T, Tremblay A, Clubb F. Endocardial hypothermia and pulmonary vein isolation with epicardial cryoablation in a porcine beating-heart model. The Journal of Thoracic and Cardiovascular Surgery. 2008;**135**:1327-1333. DOI: 10.1016/j.jtcvs.2007.12.038

[40] Schill M, Melby S, Speltz M, Breitbach M, Schuessler R, Damiano R. Evaluation of a novel Cryoprobe for atrial ablation in a chronic ovine model. The Annals of Thoracic Surgery. 2017;**104**:1069-1073. DOI: 10.1016/j.athoracsur.2017.02.041

[41] Chiappini B, Martìn-Suàrez S, LoForte A, Di Bartolomeo R, Marinelli G. Surgery for atrial fibrillation using radiofrequency catheter ablation. The Journal of Thoracic and Cardiovascular Surgery. 2003;**126**:1788-1791. DOI: 10.1016/S0022

[42] Chiappini B, Martìn-Suàrez S, LoForte A, Arpesella G, Di Bartolomeo R, Marinelli G. Cox/maze III operation versus radiofrequency ablation for the surgical treatment of atrial fibrillation: A comparative study. The Annals of Thoracic Surgery. 2004;**77**:87-92

[43] Gillinov A, Pettersson G, Rice T. Esophageal injury during radiofrequency ablation for atrial fibrillation. The Journal of Thoracic and Cardiovascular Surgery. 2001;**122**:1239-1240. DOI: 10.1067/mtc.2001.118041

[44] Yu W, Hsu T, Tai C, Tsai C, Hsieh M, Lin W, Lin Y, Tsao H, Ding Y, Chang M, Chen S. Acquired pulmonary vein stenosis after radiofrequency catheter ablation of paroxysmal atrial fibrillation. Journal of Cardiovascular Electrophysiology. 2001;**12**:887-892

[45] Bugge E, Nicholson I, Thomas S. Comparison of bipolar and unipolar radiofrequency ablation in an in vivo experimental model. European Journal of Cardio-Thoracic Surgery. 2005;**28**:76-80. DOI: 10.1016/j.ejcts.2005.02.028

[46] González-Suárez A, Trujillo M, Koruth J, d'Avila A, Berjano E. Radiofrequency cardiac ablation with catheters placed on opposing sides of the ventricular wall: Computer modelling comparing bipolar and unipolar modes. International Journal of Hyperthermia. 2014;**30**:372-384. DOI: 10.3109/02656736.2014.949878

[47] Viola N, Williams M, Oz M, Ad N. The technology in use for the surgical ablation of atrial fibrillation. Seminars in Thoracic and Cardiovascular Surgery. 2002;**14**:198-205

[48] Aupperle H, Doll N, Walther T, Ullmann C, Schoon H, Wilhelm Mohr F. Histological findings induced by different energy sources in experimental atrial ablation in sheep. Interactive Cardiovascular and Thoracic Surgery. 2005;**4**:450-455. DOI: 10.1510/icvts.2005.109413

[49] Ba M, Fornés P, Nutu O, Latrémouille C, Carpentier A, Chachques J. Treatment of atrial fibrillation by surgical epicardial ablation: Bipolar radiofrequency versus cryoablation. Archives of Cardiovascular Diseases. 2008;**101**:763-768. DOI: 10.1016/j.acvd.2008.07.004

[50] Gaynor S, Ishii Y, Diodato M, Prasad S, Barnett K, Damiano N, Byrd G, Wickline S, Schuessler R, Damiano R. Successful performance of Cox-maze procedure on beating heart using bipolar radiofrequency ablation: A feasibility study in animals. The Annals of Thoracic Surgery. 2004;**78**:1671-1677. DOI: 10.1016/j.athoracsur.2004.04.058

[51] Prasad S, Maniar H, Diodato M, Schuessler R, Damiano R. Physiological consequences of bipolar radiofrequency energy on the atria and pulmonary veins: A chronic animal study. The Annals of Thoracic Surgery. 2003;**76**:836-841

[52] Prasad S, Maniar H, Schuessler R, Damiano R. Chronic transmural atrial ablation by using bipolar radiofrequency energy on the beating heart. The Journal of Thoracic and Cardiovascular Surgery. 2002;**124**:708-713

[53] Kasirajan V, Sayeed S, Filler E, Knarik A, Koneru J, Ellenbogen K. Histopathology of bipolar radiofrequency ablation in the human atrium. The Annals of Thoracic Surgery. 2016;**101**:638-643. DOI: 10.1016/j.athoracsur.2015.07.027

[54] Kato W, Usui A, Oshima H, Akita T, Ueda Y. Incomplete transmural ablation caused by bipolar radiofrequency ablation devices. The Journal of Thoracic and Cardiovascular Surgery. 2009;**137**:251-252. DOI: 10.1016/j.jtcvs.2008.03.004

[55] Deneke T, Khargi K, Müller K, Lemke B, Mügge A, Laczkovics A, Becker A, Grewe P. Histopathology of intraoperatively induced linear radiofrequency ablation lesions in patients with chronic atrial fibrillation. European Heart Journal. 2005;**26**:1797-1803. DOI: 10.1093/eurheartj/ehi255

[56] Wakasa S, Kubota S, Shingu Y, Kato H, Ooka T, Tachibana T, Matsui Y. Histological assessment of transmurality after repeated radiofrequency ablation of the left atrial wall. General Thoracic and Cardiovascular Surgery. 2014;**62**:428-433. DOI: 10.1007/s11748-013-0363-9

[57] Gillinov A, McCarthy P. Atricure bipolar radiofrequency clamp for intraoperative ablation of atrial fibrillation. The Annals of Thoracic Surgery. 2002;**74**:2165-2168

[58] Ventosa-Fernández G, Sandoval E, Ninot S, Ribalta T, Castellá M. Histologic evidence of Transmurality four years after bipolar radiofrequency cox-maze IV. The Annals of Thoracic Surgery. 2015;**100**:328. DOI: 10.1016/j.athoracsur.2015.02.126

3

Drug Abuse-Induced Cardiac Arrhythmias: Mechanisms and Management

Sana Ouali, Omar Guermazi, Fatma Guermazi,
Manel Ben Halima, Selim Boudiche,
Nadim Khedher, Fathia Meghaieth,
Abdeljalil Farhati, Noureddine Larbi and
Mohamed Sami Mourali

Abstract

Toxicomania is a worldwide emerging problem threatening young population. Several reports highlighted its hazardous cardiovascular effects. Sudden cardiac death secondary to cardiac arrhythmias is the most occupying issue. Different forms of cardiac rhythm disorders may be induced by illicit drug abuse according to the type of drug and the mechanism involved. In this review, we exposed the main ventricular and supraventricular arrhythmia complicating the common recreational drugs, and we explained their different mechanisms as well as the particularities of management.

Keywords: cardiac arrhythmias, illicit drugs, management, mechanism

1. Introduction

Toxicomania is a worldwide health and social problem. In 2015, the World Health Organization estimates that 255 millions of people are drug users and more than 10% of them have health disorders [1]. In Tunisia, the issue is more complicated as drug abuse begins at a very early age, affecting 4.2% of students aged between 15 and 17 years old [2]. This finding results in a chronic use and a more accumulation of these substances leading to serious health complications, among which cardiovascular ones are the most occupying mainly acute coronary syndromes and rhythm disturbances resulting in more and more reported young's sudden cardiac deaths [3].

Most of the researches have focused on mental health effects and neurotoxicity of illicit drugs. Some of them were interested to cardiovascular dangers in general, and they were almost cases or series reports. The current review will focus on the topic of cardiac arrhythmias secondary to drug abuse in which we will explain their different mechanisms and principles of management.

2. Cocaine

This "white powder," extracted from coca leaves, is not only one of the oldest known stimulants but also the most known cardiotoxic illicit drug.

Several cases and series of sudden death, in the hours following cocaine consumption, were reported. The main likely cause is cocaine-induced arrhythmia [3].

Four mechanisms are implicated in the genesis of arrhythmia in case of cocaine intoxication: sodium channel blockade, potassium channel blockade, catecholamine excess, and finally myocardial infarction (MI) and myocarditis [4]. Recently, sinus bradycardia has been described as a result of chronic cocaine use [5–7] that may be related to a cocaine-induced desensitization of beta-adrenergic receptors [6].

The main measure for patients suffering from cocaine-induced arrhythmia is withholding the drug and referring to a detoxification center to prevent recurrent events. In addition, specific strategies should also be conducted according to the type of arrhythmia.

2.1. Sodium channel blockade

- Wide QRS tachycardia related to sodium channel blockade and reentry ventricular tachycardia

First, the blockade of fast inward sodium channels by cocaine is well described as a class IC effect according to the Vaughan-Williams classification of antiarrhythmic agents. Modulators of the effect of cocaine are increased in heart rate and decreased in pH which increases the degree of sodium channel blockade [8].

Electrocardiographic (ECG) manifestations mimic those of other sodium channel blockers, drugs and toxins, as tricyclic antidepressants. These manifestations depend on the degree of intoxication. In fact, early and minimal toxicity results in the impairment of conduction on the right side leading to a rightward axis deviation and QRS duration prolongation, and then, as toxicity increases, a right bundle branch block (RBBB) appears in the precordial leads (**Figure 1**). This pattern associated with sinus tachycardia, often shown in case of cocaine intoxication, may be confused with a true ventricular tachycardia resulting from a reentry or focal mechanism that can also complicate cocaine intoxication as reported in many series [4, 9, 10].

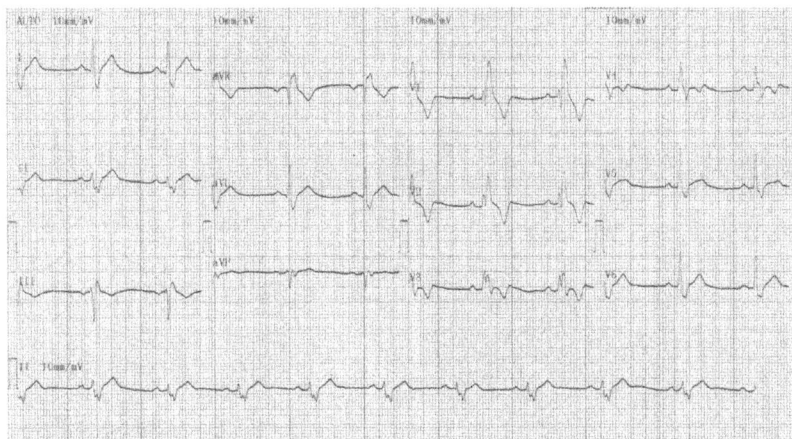

Figure 1. ECG performed after a wide QRS tachycardia cardioversion showing a complete right bundle branch block in a 38-year-old man with 10 years use of cocaine.

To manage this wide QRS tachycardia related to sodium channel blockade, general measures should rapidly be initiated. Oxygenation and ventilation should be optimized, and rapid cooling should be initiated when extreme hyperthermia is present. Sedation with a benzodiazepine is indicated to control behavior, to lower heart rate which may be sufficient to improve conduction and for its antianginal effects in patients with cocaine-associated acute coronary syndrome [4, 11].

This electrocardiographic manifestation, occurring in case of acute intoxication and mediated by pH decrease, is reversed by hypertonic sodium bicarbonate [8, 12, 13]. In case of persistence of this tachycardia with abnormal QRS prolongation, antiarrhythmic drugs should be administrated. Class IA and class IC antiarrhythmic drugs are classically contraindicated as they may potentiate QRS enlargement via a synergistic action on sodium channels. In contrast, lidocaine (class IB) can compete with cocaine for binding to the sodium channel, and it has a rapid offset responsible for the decrease in QRS duration. However, it was suggested that lidocaine exacerbated cocaine-associated seizures and arrhythmias as a result of similar effects on sodium channels [14]. Beta-blockers are contraindicated in case of cocaine intoxication as they exacerbate coronary vasospasm resulting in an increased risk of myocardial infarction [11]. No data exist concerning the efficacy of amiodarone in clinical cocaine intoxication [11].

- Brugada-like pattern

Moreover, a classic Brugada pattern has been noted in cocaine users, as seen with class IA antiarrhythmic drugs [15, 16]. It is quite likely that these patients express a sodium channel mutation described in association with Brugada abnormality and that the sodium channel blocking properties of cocaine made the patients' underlying physiological abnormality more evident [4]. Recently, El Mazloum et al. reported four cases of out-of-hospital cardiac arrest after acute cocaine intoxication associated with Brugada ECG patterns [17].

Cocaine abuse should be stopped. Mostly, ECG reverts toward normal as toxicity resolves [13]. Otherwise, sudden cardiac death risk should be evaluated, and implantable cardioverter defibrillator should be discussed in coordination with cardiac electrophysiologists.

2.2. Potassium channel blockade

Cocaine is known to block the rectifying potassium channels resulting in QT interval prolongation and hyperpolarization leading to early and late afterdepolarizations. If an afterdepolarization of significant magnitude occurs at a time when a critical number of cells can conduct an impulse, an ectopic beat can trigger a reentrant rhythm, and monomorphic ventricular tachycardia or torsades de pointes (TdP) occur [18–21].

Management of TdP and QT prolongation resulting from cocaine-associated potassium channel blockade is similar to those from other causes. In fact, for QT prolongation, electrolytic abnormalities, mainly hypokalemia and hypomagnesaemia, should be identified and rapidly corrected. Prophylactic magnesium is also suggested in patients with QT interval above 500 ms [4]. In case of TdP, magnesium, potassium replacement, and even overdrive are the main treatments. QT prolonging drugs should be withheld [4, 22].

2.3. Catecholamine excess

The common acute effect of cocaine is to block the presynaptic uptake of dopamine, norepinephrine, and epinephrine, resulting in an augmented level of these neurotransmitters at the postsynaptic terminal, producing an exaggerated catecholamine effect [23–25].

This produces sinus tachycardia, a very common finding in these patients, reentrant supraventricular tachycardia [26], and atrial fibrillation, noted in case and series reports [27].

Supportive care is generally sufficient to control sinus tachycardia. Sedation with benzodiazepine, oxygen, cooling, and volume resuscitation are the main measures. For reentrant supraventricular tachycardia, the use of a calcium channel blocker is often required. Finally, atrial fibrillation should be classically treated, using short-acting drugs as rhythm is generally controlled when toxicity resolves and avoiding β-blockers and class IA and IC antiarrhythmic drugs [4].

2.4. Myocardial infarction and myocarditis

The risk of myocardial infarction is multiplied by 24 within the next hour following cocaine consumption [28]. Cocaine-associated myocardial ischemia and infarction is a multifactorial process that results from increased demand, vasospasm, enhanced coagulation, impaired thrombolysis, and accelerated atherogenesis [29]. A catecholamine excess (trigger) induced by cocaine on such a vulnerable myocardium (substrate) may provoke the development of ventricular arrhythmias and sudden cardiac death.

In addition to myocardial infarction, scar-related macroreentrant ventricular tachycardia may also complicate cocaine-induced acute toxic myocarditis (**Figure 2**) as demonstrated in several case and series reports [30–32].

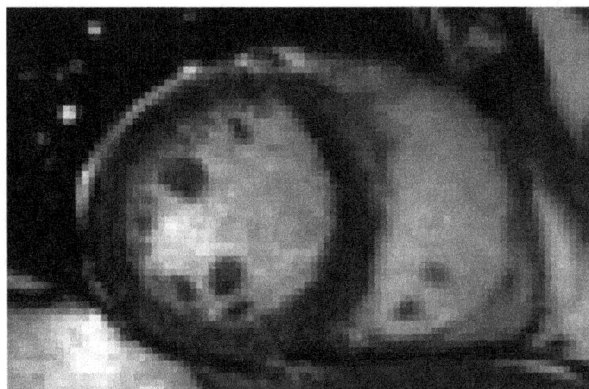

Figure 2. Cardiac magnetic resonance imaging revealing a late gadolinium enhancement (LGE) of the subepicardial layers of the septal and lateral walls of the left ventricle in a cocaine abuse man admitted for a ventricular tachycardia management.

When a cocaine-associated acute myocardial infarction is diagnosed, classical antithrombotic therapies should be administrated according to current guidelines, and primary PCI should be rapidly performed. Moreover, benzodiazepine should be initiated, and β-blockers have to be avoided because of the risk of further vasospasm [11, 33].

For scar-related reentry, as well as focal, ventricular tachycardia, management is based on classical measures and therapies according to current guidelines [34] with respect of the above-cited particularities and contraindications related to cocaine intoxication. In addition, implantable cardioverter defibrillator implantation should be deferred until the resolution of the acute episode [32, 34].

Besides these therapies, radiofrequency ablation using 3D mapping was described to be an effective therapy in 86% of drug refractory ventricular tachycardia related to cocaine use [10].

2.5. Sinus bradycardia and early repolarization pattern

Recent reports have demonstrated that chronic cocaine use is a strong predictor of sinus bradycardia compared with a matched group of nonusers and resulted in three- to seven-fold increased risk of sinus bradycardia [5–7]. Despite the presence of sinus bradycardia, all patients were able to augment their sinus rate with activity [6].

Sharma et al. have showed also that current cocaine dependence corresponds to an increased odd of demonstrating early repolarization by a factor of 4.92 [5].

Common physiological manifestations of cocaine are related to its adrenergic effects. However, with chronic exposure to cocaine, Franklin et al. have postulated that the mechanism of sinus bradycardia may be related to a cocaine-induced desensitization of beta-adrenergic receptors.

A blockage of the fast sodium current reduces sinus node automaticity, and results in brady-cardia have also been evocated [6].

3. Cannabis

Because of its accessibility and legality of use in many countries, cannabis, also known as "marijuana" or "hashish," is the most consumed drug in Tunisia and all over the world [1, 2]. Cardiovascular complications of cannabis use rose from 1.1 to 3.6% between 2006 and 2010 among 9936 abusers according to the French Addictovigilance Network, most of them presenting with an acute coronary syndrome, while two patients had cardiac arrhythmia [35]. Due to its widespread use and of possible harmful cardiovascular impact reported in many case and series reports, cardiologists should be sensitized to detect its potential dangerous effects and be able to prevent and manage them properly.

Cannabis is rapidly absorbed through the lungs and less so with ingestion. The effects of the drug can last up to 6 hours with the onset of arrhythmias beginning anywhere from within a few minutes to a few hours of smoking and with a peak at 30 minutes [36].

Delta-9-tétrahydrocannabinol (Δ-9-THC), the active agent of cannabis, exercises its action via the cannabinoid system with its two receptors CB1 and CB2. This system induces modifications of the regulation of the autonomic nervous system leading to cardiovascular consequences and of central nervous system resulting in psychoneurological effects [37, 38].

Most published reports have focused on incidents of acute coronary syndromes and acute cerebrovascular and peripheral vascular events. However, an increasing number of case reports indicate an association between cannabis use and cardiac arrhythmias mainly atrial fibrillation (AF) and ventricular arrhythmias (**Figure 3**) [39]. Management and reversibility of these arrhythmias are similar to those induced by cocaine abuse and will not be re-explained in this chapter.

In fact, cannabis has a biphasic effect on the autonomic nervous system.

3.1. Increase in sympathetic activity

At low to moderate doses, THC leads to an increase in sympathetic activity causing sinus tachycardia with a rise of 20–100% of the heart rate, premature ventricular beats associated with increased cardiac output and hypertension [36]. The concept of sympathetic activation is supported by studies demonstrating an increased urinary excretion of epinephrine after THC use [40].

Atrial fibrillation is another complication of acute cannabis intoxication. A recent study focused on causes of atrial fibrillation in young people ≤45 years old. Among 88 patients, 22 of them, the atrial fibrillation was directly related to alcohol (86.4%), cannabis (13.6%), or cocaine abuse (4.5%) [41]. In a systematic review published in 2008, six reported cases were analyzed. In all instances, AF was of recent onset occurring shortly after marijuana smoking in young subjects. No patient had a structural heart disease, and only one had a precipitating factor (hypertension); all patients had a favorable outcome with no recurrence after cessation of marijuana smoking [42]. Of note, adrenergic stimulation and disturbances in atrial coronary or microvascular flow associated with marijuana smoking may facilitate AF development and perpetuation possibly because of increased pulmonary vein ectopy, enhanced atrial electrical remodeling, and increased dispersion of refractoriness [42]. It should also be stressed that although this adverse event seems to be quite "benign" in young healthy subjects, it is apparently more "malignant" in older patients having other risk factors for thromboembolism.

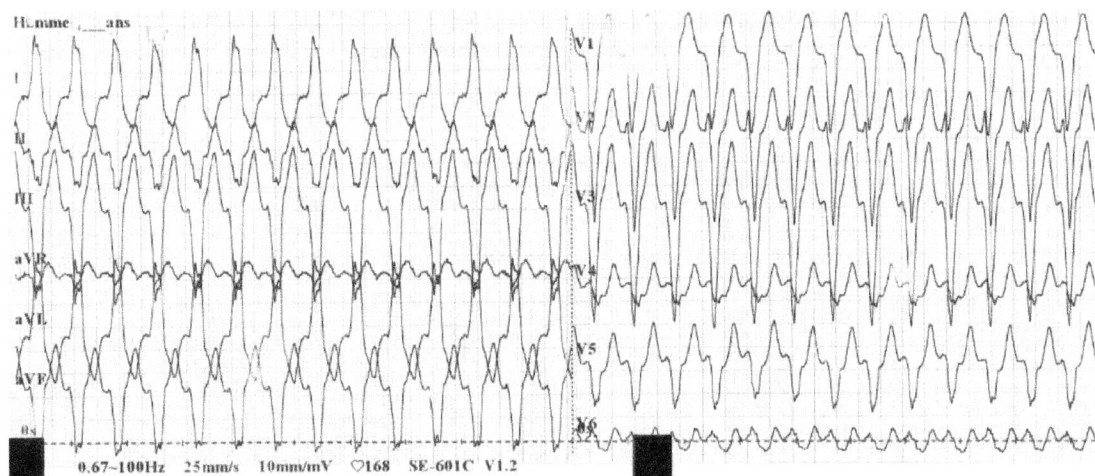

Figure 3. ECG showing a ventricular tachycardia at 170 beats/min with left bundle branch block pattern and left QRS axis in a 39-year-old man with a history of chronic cannabis use.

Finally, we should note that the burden of this problem is possibly underestimated given euphoric and neuropsychological effects of marijuana that may cover palpitations, possible occurrence of unnoticed short episodes of AF and because of social and legal reasons leading most users of illicit drugs to avoid seeking medical attention [43]. AF onset in young patients without structural heart disease should pay attention to an eventual illicit drug abuse. Its identification is very important because drug cessation will protect against AF recurrences.

3.2. Increase in parasympathetic activity

In contrast, at higher doses, parasympathetic activity is increased causing bradycardia and hypotension [36].

Bradyarrhythmias such as sinus bradycardia and higher-degree atrioventricular block have been reported. And, these conduction disturbances were reversible 72 hours after drug cessation [44].

The most described parasympathetic complication of cannabis abuse is vasovagal and postural syncope leading in some cases to sinus asystole. In a randomized controlled trial where 29 volunteers had participated, the effects of THC infusion and marijuana smoking when reclining and standing were studied. Both THC and marijuana-induced postural dizziness, with 28% reporting severe symptoms immediately after drug administration. The severe dizziness group showed the most marked postural drop in cerebral blood velocity and blood pressure and showed a drop in pulse rate after an initial increase during standing [45, 46].

3.3. Acute coronary syndrome

The risk of myocardial infarction (MI) is 4.8-fold increased in the first hour following marijuana use [47]. Urgent coronary angiography practiced in these victims of cannabis-induced MI may show angiographically normal coronary arteries supposing a spastic mechanism or an increased myocardial oxygen demand due to increased sympathetic activity. Coronary arteries may also be very thrombotic with or without atherosclerotic plaque rupture. Finally, a no-flow or slow-flow with normal appearing epicardial vessels was reported as well [48]. Ventricular tachycardia and sudden cardiac death were reported as a complication of cannabis-induced MI [49].

3.4. Sodium channel blockade

A Brugada-like effect was reported to be associated to cannabis intoxication as described with cocaine abuse [50–52]. This ECG pattern is believed to be related to a partial sodium channel antagonist activity. The ST segment normalizes once the acute intoxication is resolved.

4. Amphetamines and derivatives: ecstasy and methamphetamines

These synthetic drugs are used for their psychostimulant effects. They had been first used by German army during the Second World War for these sought effects. Later, their cardiovascular dangers were revealed.

The main mechanism of action is an indirect sympathomimetic effect by releasing norepinephrine, dopamine, and serotonin from central and autonomic nervous system terminals, leading, as in cocaine intoxication, to an increase in the central and peripheral catecholamine concentrations [53].

High catecholamine levels are known to be cardiotoxic, causing vasospasm, tachycardia, and hypertension, leading to increased myocardial oxygen demand and myocyte necrosis and fibrosis [54].

The association of these stimulants and sudden cardiac death is well established. A recent histopathological study showed that among 100 methamphetamine poisoning-related deaths, 68% had cardiac lesions [55]. In this context, death can result either from lethal aortic dissection or from ventricular arrhythmia. This latter may complicate either type 1 and type 2 myocardial infarctions or methamphetamine-induced cardiomyopathy and is triggered by catecholamine excess [56]. Furthermore, according to an interesting recent study, among 230 amphetamine abuser patients, 43% presented with sinus tachycardia and 3.5% presented with cardiac arrhythmias: ventricular tachycardia, premature atrial beats, paroxysmal supraventricular tachycardia, and premature ventricular beats [57].

5. Heroine

Morphine and its semisynthetic analogue heroin are the most commonly used recreational narcotic drugs. Narcotic agents act centrally on the vasomotor center to increase parasympathetic and reduce sympathetic activity [48, 53]. These autonomic changes, combined with histamine release from mast cell degranulation, can result in bradycardia and hypotension [53]. Sinus bradycardia, benign atrioventricular block, and resulting atrial or ventricular automatic ectopy and tachycardia were all reported. ECGs of 511 opioid addicts were analyzed. The main anomalies detected were sinus bradycardia, type-1 atrioventricular block, wandering atrial pacemaker, supraventricular and ventricular ectopic beats, and QT prolongation [58].

Methadone is another synthetic opioid used for the treatment of opioid addiction and for its analgesic effect. Methadone is responsible for QT prolongation and occurrence of torsade de pointes (TdP) especially when QT interval exceeds 500 ms. TdP should always be suspected in patients receiving methadone and presenting with syncope [59, 60]. Correction of predisposing factors as hypokalemia and hypomagnesemia is recommended, in case of prolonged QT and TdP. Magnesium perfusion is proposed, even in case of normal serum magnesium concentration. Alternative drugs can be used when corrected QT exceeds 500 ms [59].

6. Lysergic acid diethylamide and psilocybin

Lysergic acid diethylamide (LSD) and psilocybin "magic mushrooms" are commonly used hallucinogenic agents in developed countries. LSD is about 100 times more potent than psilocybin. Their mechanisms of action are complex and include agonist, partial agonist, and antagonist effects at various serotonin, dopaminergic, and adrenergic receptors. The adrenergic effects are usually mild and do not produce the profound sympathetic storms that can occur after taking cocaine, amphetamine, or ecstasy. Besides common sinus tachycardia, cardiovascular complications are rarely serious, although occasional instances of supraventricular tachyarrhythmias and myocardial infarction have been reported [61, 62].

7. Inhalent abuse

Inhalant abuse is the intentional inhalation of chemical vapors by sniffing, snorting, bagging, or huffing the substance to attain a euphoric effect. Spray paints, shoe polish, dust-off spray, glue, and lighter fluids are some products commonly abused by people. Glue sniffing has become a widespread form of inhalant abuse, usually among in adolescents and young adults.

Studies have indicated that about 20% of children in middle and high schools have experimented with inhalant substances [63]. These products are cheap, easily accessible at home, school, and workplace, and they are legal for all age groups (e.g., glue). Many common household products containing halogenated hydrocarbon like 1,1-difluoroethane (DFE) (known as Freon 152A used in refrigeration, dust-off spray, and airbrush painting) and toluene (used in glues) are abused by inhalation for euphoric effects [64].

Halogenated hydrocarbon abuse can cause a fatal malignant arrhythmia, termed "sudden sniffing death." Cardiotoxic effects have been described in human and in animal models [64].

Avella et al. [65] have demonstrated different levels in DFE tissues in the brain and heart, but the DFE level in the heart remained higher than the brain tissue after approximately

60-second post-DFE withdrawal. This may further result in abuser inhaling more DFE to sustain euphoric effect because central nervous system effects are reduced and thus lead to accumulation in the heart.

Recently, Joshi et al. [66] have showed that after multiple DFE doses in rats, severe arrhythmias such as ventricular fibrillation and ventricular tachycardia can be triggered. Exposure causes significant higher amount of epinephrine release than the control group [66] and an increased sensitivity of the myocardium to epinephrine [64, 67]. Furthermore, electrolyte imbalance, cardiac biomarkers, and oxidative stress markers were significantly affected and can cause damage to cardiomyocytes [66].

Alper et al. have demonstrated increase in QT duration, QT, and QTc dispersion in toluene users [68]. Toluene can cause inhibition of cardiac sodium currents like class I antiarrhythmics which can cause prolonged QT interval and have proarrhythmic effects [69].

Although the electrical function of the heart can be altered with acute exposure to hydrocarbons, prolonged use can cause structural damage that may also impede normal function [64].

Samples of cardiac muscle taken from inhalant abusers have shown interstitial edema, intramyocardial hemorrhages, contraction band necrosis, [70] edema, swollen and ruptured myofibrils, [71] and myocarditis and interstitial fibrosis [72].

In addition to arrhythmias, halogenated hydrocarbons have negative inotropic, dromotropic, and chronotropic effects on cardiac tissue [73]. Cases of atrioventricular conduction abnormality have been described in toluene intoxication [74].

8. Conclusion

Cardiac arrhythmia presents a potential dangerous complication leading to sudden cardiac death threatening young population. The most important mechanisms implicated in the genesis of arrhythmia in case of illicit drug intoxication are sodium channel blockade, potassium channel blockade, catecholamine excess, and finally myocardial infarction and myocarditis. Atrial fibrillation onset in young patients without structural heart disease should pay attention to an eventual illicit drug abuse. Its identification is very important because drug cessation will protect against atrial fibrillation recurrences. **Table 1** resumes physiopathological effects and main induced arrhythmias of commonly abused illicit drugs. Management should consist, first, on withholding drug intoxication with the collaboration of a detoxification center to prevent recurrent events, and, second, on common recommended measures as for the treatment of nondrug abuse arrhythmias with respect of some particularities and contraindications as in the case of cocaine intoxication. Thus, acute management of wide QRS tachycardia related to sodium channel blockade secondary to drug abuse, include oxygenation, sedation with benzodiazepine, and hypertonic sodium bicarbonate perfusion. Class IA and class IC antiarrhythmic drugs and betablockers are classically contraindicated. Electrical cardioversion is indicated in case of all hemodynamically unstable arrhythmias.

Illicit drug	Physiopathological effects	Induced cardiac arrhythmias
Cocaine	Sodium channel blockade	QRS enlargement with right bundle branch block
		Brugada-like syndrome
	Potassium channel blockade	QT prolongation
		Torsade de pointes
	Catecholamine excess	Sinus tachycardia
		Supraventricular tachycardia
	Myocardial infarction/myocarditis	Ventricular tachycardia/fibrillation
	Cocaine-induced desensitization of beta-adrenergic receptors	Sinus bradycardia
Cannabis	Increase in sympathetic activity	Sinus tachycardia
		Atrial fibrillation
		Premature ventricular beats
	Increase in parasympathetic activity	Sinus bradycardia
		Atrioventricular block
		Vasovagal and postural syncope
		Sinus asystole
	Myocardial infarction	Ventricular tachycardia/fibrillation
	Sodium channel blockade	Brugada-like syndrome
Methamphetamine and ecstasy	Catecholamine excess	Sinus tachycardia
		Supraventricular tachycardia
	Myocardial infarction	Ventricular tachycardia/fibrillation
Heroine and morphine methadone	Increase parasympathetic and reduce sympathetic activity	Sinus bradycardia
		Atrial or ventricular ectopy
	Potassium channel blockade	QT prolongation
		Torsade de pointes
LSD and psilocybin	Mild catecholamine excess	Sinus tachycardia

Table 1. Physiopathological effects and main induced arrhythmias of commonly abused illicit drugs.

Conflict of interest

None declared.

Author's contribution

All authors conceived, read, and approved the final manuscript.

Author details

Sana Ouali[1]*, Omar Guermazi[1], Fatma Guermazi[2], Manel Ben Halima[1], Selim Boudiche[1], Nadim Khedher[1], Fathia Meghaieth[1], Abdeljalil Farhati[1], Noureddine Larbi[1] and Mohamed Sami Mourali[1]

*Address all correspondence to: sanaouali@hotmail.fr

1 Cardiology Department, La Rabta Hospital, Tunis, Tunisia

2 Psychiatry Department, Hedi Chaker Hospital, Sfax, Tunisia

References

[1] UNODC. Executive Summary. Conclusion and Policy Implications of the World Drug Report [Internet]. 2017. Available from: https://www.unodc.org/wdr2017/field/Booklet_1_EXSUM.pdf

[2] De S, Nationale TE. Enquête MedSPAD en Tunisie: Résultats de l'enquête nationale. 2014. Available from: https://www.coe.int/T/DG3/Pompidou/Source/Activities/MedNET/activities2014/MedSPAD-TunisieFR-V5.pdf

[3] Fischbach P. The role of illicit drug use in sudden death in the young. Cardiology in the Young. 2017;**27**(S1):S75-S79

[4] Hoffman RS. Treatment of patients with cocaine-induced arrhythmias: Bringing the bench to the bedside. British Journal of Clinical Pharmacology. 2010;**69**(5):448-457

[5] Sharma J, Rathnayaka N, Green C, Moeller FG, Schmitz JM, Shoham D, Dougherty AH. Bradycardia as a marker of chronic cocaine use: A novel cardiovascular finding. Behavioral Medicine. 2016;**42**:1e8

[6] Franklin SM, Thihalolipavan S, Fontaine JM. Sinus bradycardia in habitual cocaine users. The American Journal of Cardiology. 2017;**119**(10):1611-1615

[7] Mahoney JJ 3rd, Haile CN, De La Garza R 2nd, Thakkar H, Newton TF. Electrocardiographic characteristics in individuals with cocaine use disorder. The American Journal on Addictions. 2017;**26**(3):221-227

[8] Wang RY. pH-dependent cocaine-induced cardiotoxicity. The American Journal of Emergency Medicine. 1999;**17**(4):364-369

[9] Afonso L, Mohammad T, Thatai D. Crack whips the heart: A review of the cardiovascular toxicity of cocaine. The American Journal of Cardiology. 2007;**100**(6):1040-1043

[10] Lakkireddy D, Kanmanthareddy A, Biria M, Madhu Reddy Y, Pillarisetti J, Mahapatra S, et al. Radiofrequency ablation of drug refractory ventricular tachycardia related to cocaine use: A feasibility, safety, and efficacy study. Journal of Cardiovascular Electrophysiology. 2014;**25**(7):739-746

[11] McCord J, Jneid H, Hollander JE, De Lemos JA, Cercek B, Hsue P, et al. Management of cocaine-associated chest pain and myocardial infarction: A scientific statement from the American Heart Association acute cardiac care committee of the council on clinical cardiology. Circulation. 2008;**117**(14):1897-1907

[12] Beckman KJ, Parker RB, Hariman RJ, Gallastegui JL, Javaid JI, Bauman JL. Hemodynamic and electrophysiological actions of cocaine. Effects of sodium bicarbonate as an antidote in dogs. Circulation. 1991;**83**(5):1799-1807

[13] Winecoff AP, Hariman RJ, Grawe JJ, Wang Y, Bauman JL. Reversal of the electrocardiographic effects of cocaine by lidocaine. Part 1. Comparison with sodium bicarbonate and quinidine. Pharmacotherapy. 1994;**14**(6):704-711

[14] Derlet RW, Albertson TE, Tharratt RS. Lidocaine potentiation of cocaine toxicity. Annals of Emergency Medicine. 1991;**20**(2):135-138

[15] Littmann L, Monroe MH, Svenson RH. Brugada-type electrocardiographic pattern induced by cocaine. Mayo Clinic Proceedings. 2000;**75**(8):845-849

[16] Bebarta VS, Summers S. Brugada electrocardiographic pattern induced by cocaine toxicity. Annals of Emergency Medicine. 2007;**49**(6):827-829

[17] El Mazloum R, Snenghi R, Zorzi A, Zilio F, Dorigo A, Montisci R, Corrado D, Montisci M. Out-of-hospital cardiac arrest after acute cocaine intoxication associated with Brugada ECG patterns: Insights into physiopathologic mechanisms and implications for therapy. International Journal of Cardiology. 2015;**195**:245-249

[18] Singh N, Singh HK, Singh PP, Khan IA. Cocaine-induced torsades de pointes in idiopathic long Q-T syndrome. American Journal of Therapeutics. 2001;**8**(4):299-302

[19] Kimura S, Bassett AL, Xi H, Myerburg RJ. Early afterdepolarizations and triggered activity induced by cocaine. A possible mechanism of cocaine arrhythmogenesis. Circulation. 1992;**85**(6):2227-2235

[20] Perera R, Kraebber A, Schwartz MJ. Prolonged QT interval and cocaine use. Journal of Electrocardiology. 1997;**30**(4):337-339

[21] Riaz K, McCullough PA. Fatal case of delayed repolarization due to cocaine abuse and global ischemia. Reviews in Cardiovascular Medicine. 2003;**4**(1):47-53

[22] Sorajja D, Munger TM, Shen W-K. Optimal antiarrhythmic drug therapy for electrical storm. The Journal of Biomedical Research. 2015;**29**(1):20-34

[23] Vongpatanasin W, Mansour Y, Chavoshan B, et al. Cocaine stimulates the human cardiovascular system via a central mechanism of action. Circulation. 1999;**100**:497-502

[24] Sofuoglu M, Nelson D, Babb DA, et al. Intravenous cocaine increases plasma epinephrine and norepinephrine in humans. Pharmacology, Biochemistry, and Behavior. 2001;**68**:455-459

[25] Lange RA, Hills LD. Cardiovascular complications of cocaine use. The New England Journal of Medicine. 2001;**345**:351-358

[26] Chakko S, Sepulveda S, Kessler KM, Sotomayor MC, Mash DC, Prineas RJ, et al. Frequency and type of electrocardiographic abnormalities in cocaine abusers (electrocardiogram in cocaine abuse). The American Journal of Cardiology. 1994;**74**(7):710-713

[27] Merigian KS. Cocaine-induced ventricular arrhythmias and rapid atrial fibrillation temporally related to naloxone administration. The American Journal of Emergency Medicine. 1993;**11**(1):96-97

[28] Mittleman MA, Mintzer D, Maclure M, Tofler GH, Sherwood JB, Muller JE. Triggering of myocardial infarction by cocaine. Circulation. 1999;**99**(21):2737-2741

[29] Talarico GP, Crosta ML, Giannico MB, Summaria F, Calò L, Patrizi R. Cocaine and coronary artery diseases: A systematic review of the literature. Journal of Cardiovascular Medicine (Hagerstown, Md.). 2017;**18**(5):291-294

[30] Rijal S, Cavalcante JL. Acute cocaine myocarditis: A word of caution. European Heart Journal. 2015;**36**(15):946

[31] Virmani R, Robinowitz M, Smialek JE, Smyth DF. Cardiovascular effects of cocaine: An autopsy study of 40 patients. American Heart Journal. 1988;**115**(5):1068-1076

[32] Caforio ALP, Pankuweit S, Arbustini E, Basso C, Gimeno-Blanes J, Felix SB, et al. Current state of knowledge on aetiology, diagnosis, management, and therapy of myocarditis: A position statement of the European Society of Cardiology Working Group on myocardial and pericardial diseases. European Heart Journal. 2013;**34**(33):2636-2648

[33] Ibanez B, James S, Agewall S, Antunes MJ, Bucciarelli-Ducci C, Bueno H, Caforio ALP, Crea F, Goudevenos JA, Halvorsen S, Hindricks G, Kastrati A, Lenzen MJ, Prescott E, Roffi M, Valgimigli M, Varenhorst C, Vranckx P, Widimský P. ESC Scientific Document Group. 2017 ESC Guidelines for the management of acute myocardial infarction in patients presenting with ST-segment elevation: The Task Force for the management of acute myocardial infarction in patients presentingwith ST-segment elevation of the European Society of Cardiology (ESC). European Heart Journal. 2018;**39**(2):119-177

[34] Priori SG, Blomström-Lundqvist C, Mazzanti A, Blom N, Borggrefe M, Camm J, et al. 2015 ESC guidelines for the management of patients with ventricular arrhythmias and the prevention of sudden cardiac death. European Heart Journal. 2015;**36**(41):2793-2867

[35] Jouanjus E, Lapeyre-Mestre M, Micallef J. Cannabis use: Signal of increasing risk of serious cardiovascular disorders. Journal of the American Heart Association. 2014;**3**(2):1-7

[36] Johnson S, Domino EF. Some cardiovascular effects of marihuana smoking in normal volunteers. Clinical Pharmacology and Therapeutics. 1971;**12**(5):762-768

[37] Bouccin E, Eloye H, Hantson P. Complications vasculaires périphériques, cardiaques et cérébrales associeés à l'utilisation du cannabis. Annals of Clinical Toxicology. 2016;**28**(2):115-128

[38] Jones RT. Cardiovascular system effects of marijuana. Journal of Clinical Pharmacology. 2002;**42**:58S-63S

[39] Thomas G, Kloner RA, Rezkalla S. Adverse cardiovascular, cerebrovascular, and peripheral vascular effects of marijuana inhalation: What cardiologists need to know. The American Journal of Cardiology. 2014;**113**(1):187-190

[40] Weiss JL, Watanabe AM, Lemberger L, Tamarkin NR, Cardon PV. Cardiovascular effects of delta-9-tetrahydrocannabinol in man. Clinical Pharmacology and Therapeutics. 1972;**13**(5):671-684

[41] Krishnamoorthy S, Lip GYH, Lane DA. Alcohol and illicit drug use as precipitants of atrial fibrillation in young adults: A case series and literature review. The American Journal of Medicine. 2009;**122**(9):851-856.e3

[42] Korantzopoulos P, Liu T, Papaioannides D, Li G, Goudevenos JA. Atrial fibrillation and marijuana smoking. International Journal of Clinical Practice. 2008;**62**(2):308-313

[43] Korantzopoulos P. Marijuana smoking is associated with atrial fibrillation. The American Journal of Cardiology. 2014;**113**(6):1085-1086

[44] Akins D, Awdeh MR. Marijuana and second-degree AV block. Southern Medical Journal. 1981;**74**(3):371-373

[45] Mathew RJ, Wilson WH, Davis R. Postural syncope after marijuana: A transcranial Doppler study of the hemodynamics. Pharmacology, Biochemistry, and Behavior. 2003;**75**(2):309-318

[46] Brancheau D, Blanco J, Gholkar G, Patel B, Machado C. Cannabis induced asystole. Journal of Electrocardiology. 2016;**49**(1):15-17

[47] Mittleman MA, Lewis RA, Maclure M, Sherwood JB, Muller JE. Triggering myocardial infarction by marijuana. Circulation. 2001;**103**(23):2805-2809

[48] Harbaoui B. Complications cardiovasculaires de la toxicomanie. Archives des Maladies du Coeur et des Vaisseaux – Pratique. 2017;**256**:11-18

[49] Rezkalla SH, Sharma P, Kloner RA. Coronary no-flow and ventricular tachycardia associated with habitual marijuana use. Annals of Emergency Medicine. 2003;**42**(3):365-369

[50] Romero-Puche AJ, Trigueros-Ruiz N, Cerdan-Sanchez MC, Perez-Lorente F, Roldan D, Vicente-Vera T. Brugada electrocardiogram pattern induced by cannabis. Revista Española de Cardiología (English Edition). 2012;**65**(9):856-858

[51] Daccarett M, Freih M, Machado C. Acute cannabis intoxication mimicking brugada-like ST segment abnormalities. International Journal of Cardiology. 2007;**119**(2):235-236

[52] Pratap B, Korniyenko A. Toxic effects of marijuana on the cardiovascular system. Cardiovascular Toxicology. 2012;**12**(2):143-148

[53] Ghuran A, Nolan J. The cardiac complications of recreational drug use. The Western Journal of Medicine. 2000;**173**(6):412-415

[54] Karch's SBK. Pathology of Drug Abuse. 3rd ed. Boca Raton: CRC Press; 2002

[55] Akhgari M, Mobaraki H, Etemadi-Aleagha A. Histopathological study of cardiac lesions in methamphetamine poisoning-related deaths. Daru. 2017;25(1):5

[56] Kaye S, McKetin R, Duflou J, Darke S. Methamphetamine and cardiovascular pathology: A review of the evidence. Addiction. 2007;102(8):1204-1211

[57] Bazmi E, Mousavi F, Giahchin L, Mokhtari T, Behnoush B. Cardiovascular complications of acute amphetamine abuse: Cross-sectional study. Sultan Qaboos University Medical Journal. 2017;17(1):e31-e37

[58] Wallner C, Stöllberger C, Hlavin A, Finsterer J, Hager I, Hermann P. Electrocardiographic abnormalities in opiate addicts. Addiction. 2008;103(12):1987-1993

[59] Alinejad S, Kazemi T, Zamani N, Hoffman RS, Mehrpour O. A systematic review of the cardiotoxicity of methadone. EXCLI Journal. 2015;14:577-600

[60] Fanoe S, Hvidt C, Ege P, Jensen GB. Syncope and QT prolongation among patients treated with methadone for heroin dependence in the city of Copenhagen. Heart. 2007;93(9): 1051-1055

[61] Borowiak KS, Ciechanowski K, Waloszczyk P. Psilocybin mushroom (Psilocybe semilanceata) intoxication with myocardial infarction. Journal of Toxicology. Clinical Toxicology. 1998;36(1-2):47-49

[62] Ghuran A. Recreational drug misuse: Issues for the cardiologist. Heart. 2000;83(6):627-633

[63] U.S. Department of Health and Human Services. Monitoring the future survey release. Smoking among teenagers decreases sharply and increase in ecstasy use slows. U.S. Department of Health and Human Services HHS News; December 19; 2001. Retrieved July 3, 2003, from: www.nida.nih.gov/MedAdv/01/NR12-19.html

[64] Tormoehlen LM, Tekulve KJ, Nañagas KA. Hydrocarbon toxicity: A review. Clinical Toxicology (Philadelphia, Pa.). 2014;52:479-489

[65] Avella J, Kunaparaju N, Kumar S, et al. Uptake and distribution of the abused inhalant 1,1-difluoroethane in the rat. Journal of Analytical Toxicology. 2010;34:381-388

[66] Joshi K, Barletta M, Wurpel J. Cardiotoxic (Arrhythmogenic) effects of 1,1-difluoroethane due to electrolyte imbalance and cardiomyocyte damage. The American Journal of Forensic Medicine and Pathology. 2017;38(2):115-125

[67] Himmel HM. Mechanisms involved in cardiac sensitization by volatile anesthetics: General applicability to halogenated hydrocarbons? Critical Reviews in Toxicology. 2008;38:773-803

[68] Alper AT, Akyol A, Hasdemir H, Nurkalem Z, Güler O, Güvenç TS, Erdinler I, Cakmak N, Eksik A, Gürkan K. Glue (toluene) abuse: Increased QT dispersion and relation with unexplained syncope. Inhalation Toxicology. 2008;20(1):37-41

[69] Cruz SL, Orta-Salazar G, Gauthereau MY, et al. Inhibition of cardiac sodium currents by toluene exposure. British Journal of Pharmacology. 2003;140:653-660

[70] Sakai K, Maruyama-Maebashi K, Takatsu A, Fukui K, Nagai T, Aoyagi M, et al. Sudden death involving inhalation of 1,1-difluoroethane (HFC-152a) with spray cleaner: Three case reports. Forensic Science International. 2011;**206**:e58-e61

[71] Banathy LJ, Chan LT. Fatality caused by inhalation of "liquid paper" correction fluid. The Medical Journal of Australia. 1983;**2**(12):606

[72] Wiseman MN, Banim S. "Glue sniffer's" heart? British Medical Journal (Clinical Research Ed.). 1987;**294**(6574):739

[73] Muller SP, Wolna P, Wunscher U, Pankow D. Cardiotoxicity of chlorodibromomethane and trichloromethane in rats and isolated rat cardiac myocytes. Archives of Toxicology. 1997;**71**:766-777

[74] Tsao JH, Hu YH, How CK, Chern CH, Hung-Tsang Yen D, Huang CI. Atrioventricular conduction abnormality and hyperchloremic metabolic acidosis in toluene sniffing. Journal of the Formosan Medical Association. 2011;**110**(10):652-654

Endocardial Approach for Substrate Ablation in Brugada Syndrome

Pablo E. Tauber, Virginia Mansilla, Pedro Brugada,
Sara S. Sánchez, Stella M. Honoré, Marcelo Elizari,
Sergio Chain Molina, Felix A. Albano,
Ricardo R. Corbalán,
Federico Figueroa Castellanos and
Damian Alzugaray Bioeng

Abstract

Radiofrequency ablation (RFA) in Brugada syndrome (BrS) has been performed by both endocardial and epicardial. The substrate in BrS is not completely understood. We investigate the functional endocardial substrate and its correlation with clinical, electrophysiological and ECG findings in order to guide an endocardial ablation. Two patients agreed to undergo an endocardial biopsy and the samples were examined with transmission electron microscopy (TEM) to investigate the correlation between functional and ultrastructural alterations. About 13 patients (38.7 ± 12.3 years old) with spontaneous type 1 ECG BrS pattern, inducible VF with programmed ventricular stimulation (PVS) and syncope without prodromes were enrolled. Before endocardial mapping, the patients underwent flecainide testing with the purpose of measuring the greatest ST-segment elevation for to be correlated with the size and location of substrate in the electro-anatomic map. Patients underwent endocardial bipolar and electro-anatomic mapping with the purpose of identify areas of abnormal electrograms (EGMs) as target for RFA and determine the location and size of the substrate. When the greatest ST-segment elevation was in the third intercostal space (ICS), the substrate was located upper in the longitudinal plane of the right ventricular outflow tract (RVOT) and a greatest ST-segment elevation in fourth ICS correspond with a location of substrate in lower region of longitudinal plane of RVOT. A QRS complex widening on its initial and final part, with prolonged transmural and regional depolarization time of RVOT corresponded to the substrate located in the anterior-lateral region of RVOT. A QRS complex widening rightwards and only prolonged transmural depolarization time corresponded with a substrate located in the anterior, anterior-septal or septal region of RVOT. RFA of endocardial substrate suppressed the inducibility and ECG BrS pattern during 34.7 ± 15.5 months. After RFA, flecainide testing confirmed elimination of the ECG BrS pattern. Endocardial biopsy showed a correlation between functional and ultrastructural alterations. Endocardial RFA can eliminate the BrS phenotype and inducibility during programmed ventricular stimulation (PVS).

Keywords: Brugada syndrome, radiofrequency catheter ablation, electrocardiography, mapping, biopsy

1. Introduction

Since the original publication in 1992 [1], many researchers have tried to explain the mechanisms and substrate that causes an abnormal electrocardiographic (ECG) pattern and ventricular arrhythmias in Brugada syndrome (BrS) and few therapeutic options have been found. Initially three hypotheses were proposed for explain the mechanism and arrhythmias in BrS, the abnormal repolarization theory [2], the abnormal depolarization theory [3] and the abnormal expression of neural crest cells during cardiac development [4].

BrS is characterized by an elevated ST segment in the right precordial leads (V1–3) on the ECG and risk of sudden cardiac death (SCD) [1, 5]. The ECG 1 pattern is frequently intermittent and can be unmasked by the administration of a sodium channel blocker (**Figure 1**). The incidence of SCD in subjects with Brugada type 1 ECG pattern and no previous cardiac arrest is 2 per 1000 patients per year [6, 7].

At present, there are just two therapeutic strategies, which include implantable cardioverter-defibrillator (ICD) and/or chronic quinidine therapy [6, 7]. However, quinidine is not effective

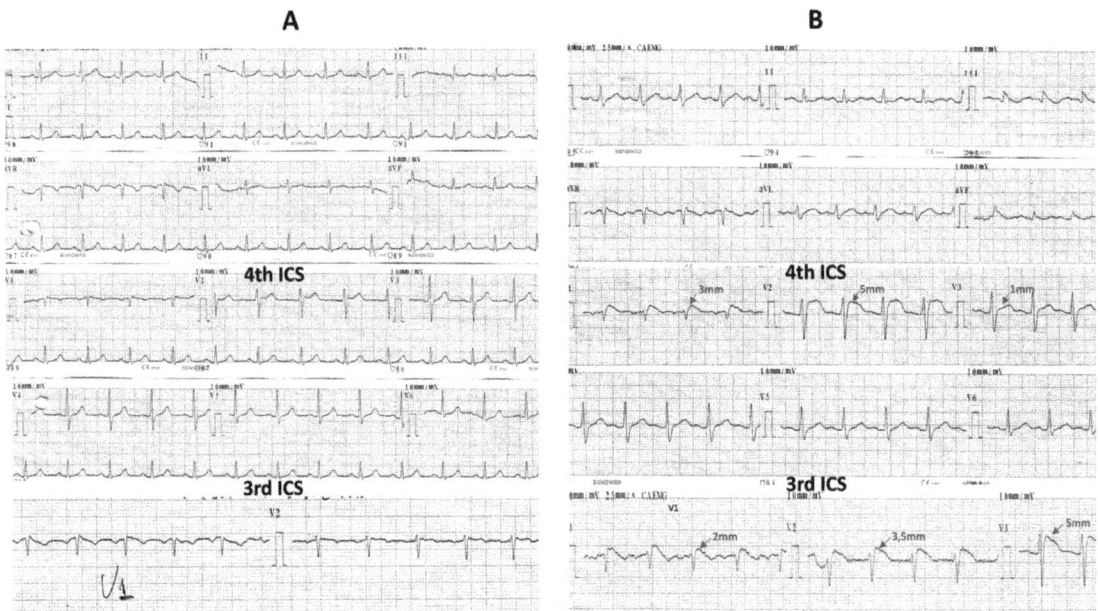

Figure 1. Characteristic BrS ECG. A. In the N°3 patient the ECG at baseline show spontaneous and intermittent type 1 ECG BrS pattern. B. After flecainide test (400 mg, orally) [19].

in many patients and its use is frequently associated with intolerable adverse effects. ICD implantation may be effective in preventing SCD, and is currently recommended as a class I indication for symptomatic patients with type 1 Brugada ECG pattern. Unfortunately, ICD therapy in many patients is associated with inappropriate shocks (overall ICD complication rate is 9.1% and inappropriate shocks in BrS occur in 13.7%), lead fractures/failure, device infections and frequent ICD discharges by electric storms [6, 8, 9].

As an autosomal dominant disease with incomplete penetrance, BrS was initially linked to mutations in the SCN5A gene [9]. Currently, more than 450 pathogenic variants have been identified in 24 genes encoding sodium, potassium, and calcium channels or associated proteins [10, 11]. Known BrS-susceptibility genes can only partially explain the clinically diagnosed cases; therefore, many patients (65–70%) remain "genetically unresolved" [8, 9]. For many years, BrS has been considered a purely electric disease even if, more recently some authors have shown the presence of morphological and functional abnormalities (regional conduction slow in the endocardium and epicardium), predominantly located in the right ventricle outflow tract (RVOT) [12–14].

Radiofrequency ablation (RFA) has recently emerged as a therapeutic option in BrS patients of high risk. RFA in two previous reports was effective in preventing ventricular fibrillation (VF) in BrS [15, 16]. Two studies have recently shown fractionated systolic electrograms (EGMs) in epicardium of RVOT and RF normalized the ECG pattern and prevented ventricular fibrillation and ventricular tachycardia (VT/VF) occurrence in a short follow-up [17, 18].

2. Study population and risk factors

The arrhythmic events occur in patients who presented spontaneous type 1 ECG BrS pattern and syncope of presumed arrhythmic origin, so both are considered high-risk factors [6]. The risk of SCD in patients without ICD is 2 per 1000 patients per year [6, 7]. But unfortunately, the possibility of survival out of hospital is low if the first symptom is the SCD.

We in a prospective single-center study consecutively included 13 caucasian patients when they presented all three high-risk criteria: (1) documented spontaneous type 1 BrS ECG pattern, (2) syncope of probable arrhythmic cause (syncope was defined as a no traumatic and reversible loss of consciousness, and was considered of arrhythmic origin in the absence of a prodrome or triggering circumstances), (3) inducible VF with PVS [19]. These were associated with at least one of the following conditions: family history of SCD at age < 45 years, type 1 BrS ECG pattern in family members, early repolarization pattern, and/or nocturnal agonal respiration [6, 9]. Structural heart disease, systemic diseases and phenocopies was ruled out in each case on the basis of clinical history and extensive evaluation with 2D Echocardiography, tilt test, brain computed tomography, 24-hour ambulatory ECG monitoring, HIV test, coxsackie and parvovirus B19 test, Chagas disease test, myocardial perfusion and cardiac nuclear magnetic resonance. All patients had 5 points according to the risk score model currently proposed by Sieira et al. [20] (spontaneous type 1 ECG pattern =1 point, inducible VF =2 points and syncope =2 points). None had a history of SCD or documented spontaneous VT/VF and did not receive antiarrhythmic drugs. Patients were submitted to endocardial bipolar and electroanatomic mapping and RFA. One month before of mapping and RFA, 10 patients accepted the implant of an ICD with class IIa indication [9]. **Table 1** shows the clinical characteristics of the study patients. About 13 patients with spontaneous type 1 ECG BrS pattern, symptomatic by syncope without prodromes, and VF induced during programed ventricular stimulation (PVS) were enrolled and completed the study protocol. Five males (38.5%) and eight females (61.5%), with an average age of 38.7 ± 12.3 years (range 19–58 years) were enrolled. Most patients (54%) had a family history of SCD and all patients experienced previous syncopal episodes without prodromes. In four patients (31%) nocturnal agonal respiration and family history of ECG 1 BrS pattern were evident. All patients had a VRP ≤ 200 m (180 ± 13.6 ms). A QRS complex duration >120 ms in V1 or V2 leads (129.6 ± 27 ms) in six patients (46%) and a R wave with an amplitude ≥3 mm in aVR lead during flecainide testing (3 ± 1.4 mm) in seven patients (54%) was found. In five patients (38.5%) a HV interval to DI lead >55 ms (53.4 ± 21 ms), in three patients a QRS fragmentation (23%) and in two patients a J wave (15.4%) were present. Interestingly, during bipolar mapping after premature ventricular contractions (PVCs), alternating T and J-wave and changes of the ST segment elevation were found (**Figure 2**).

Syncope constitutes an important diagnostic and therapeutic challenge in BrS. Approximately one-third of BrS patients present syncope. Some cases of syncope may be related to VF that terminates spontaneously. Vagal syncope is probably the most frequent cause of syncope in the BrS [21] and vagal hypertony may facilitate the onset of spontaneous VF in BrS [22]. Also symptoms suggesting of vagal syncope may also be observed in syncope of cardiac origin [23]. In our study, two patients (15%) after RFA had near-syncope with vaso-vagal prodrome and without arrhythmias in the ICD interrogation [19].

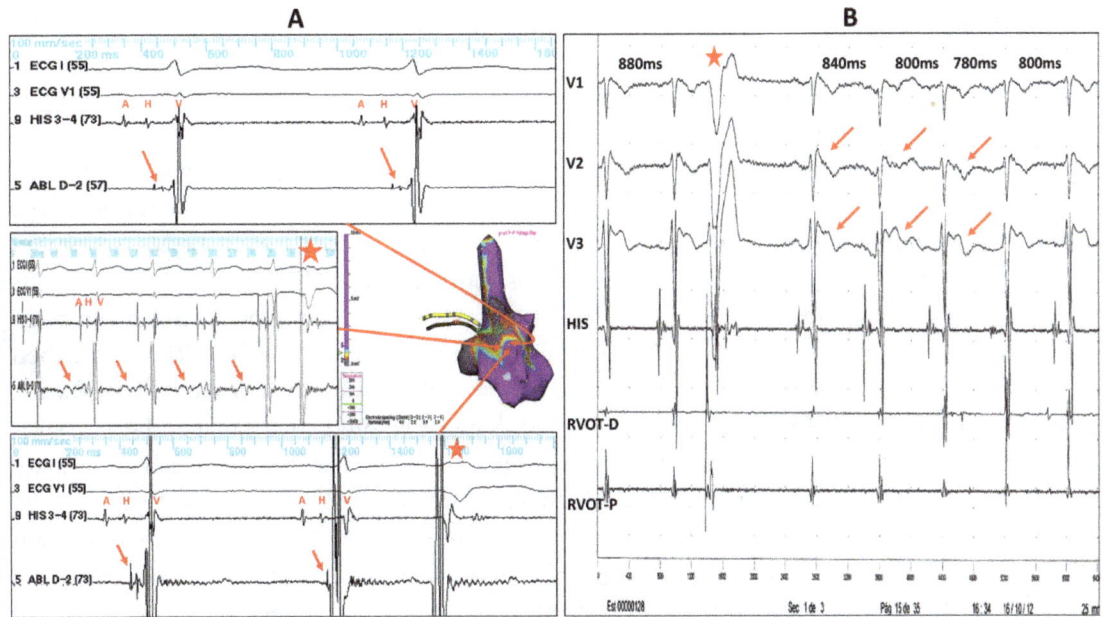

Figure 2. Endocardial mapping. A. The N° 3 patient in the peripheral zone of substrate show middle diastolic, presystolic and continuous EGMs. The split pre-systolic potential (red arrows) triggers PVC (red star). B. After PVCs (red star), alternating T and J wave are shown (electric turbulence). Also displays spontaneous ST segment elevation changes (red arrows) [19].

BrS is eight times more prevalent in males, probably for higher testosterone levels and a more prominent transient outward current (Ito). Males are at increased risk for developing a spontaneous type 1 ECG BrS pattern and VF during PVS. Nevertheless, because the majority of the asymptomatic patients are also male the gender is not an independent predictor of arrhythmic events [9, 24]. It is striking that eight of our patients (61.5%) were females. Five of these had between 38 and 58 years of age and menopausal symptoms, so we might suspect that lack of estrogens could induce the expression of phenotype [19].

3. Electrophysiological study and mapping: identification of functional substrate

Nademanee et al., found prolonged and fractionated late potentials in the anterior zone of epicardium of RVOT [17]. Recently, Brugada et al. in 14 inducible patients reported abnormal EGMs only in epicardium of the anterior free wall of right ventricle and in RVOT [18]. However, consistently we find a substrate in the endocardium of RVOT and RFA eliminates abnormal EGMs, ECG BrS pattern and inducibility during a median follow-up of 44.7 ± 15.5 months in 13 patients. We saw the substrate not only in the anterior zone of RVOT but also in septal and lateral regions, but never in the posterior region [19]. Sunsaneewitayakul et al. reported late depolarization zones on the endocardial of RVOT. Endocardial RFA about these zones modified the ECG BrS pattern and suppress the VF storm [16]. Similarly, we reported areas with late depolarization, diastolic electrical activity and abnormal systolic EGMs. In our study high-density detailed endocardial electroanatomical and bipolar voltage mapping of right ventricle and RVOT was performed, using 3-dimensional (3D) mapping system En Site NavXTM under local anesthesia and sedation, during stable sinus rhythm [19]. AH and HV interval to DI and V2 lead and ventricular refractory period (VRP) were measured. Bipolar EGMs were filtered from 10 to 400 Hz and displayed at 100–200 mm/s speeds. Systolic EGMs with an amplitude ≤1.5 Mv, split or fractionated whit a duration >80 ms and delayed components extending beyond the end of QRS complex and accompanied by late potentials (LPs) were defined as abnormal. The EGMs found in the diastole were referred as "diastolic electrical activity". The number of diastolic EGMs (separated by isoelectric line) in two successive sinus cycles was counted. PVS of RVOT with 3 cycle lengths (600, 500 and 400 ms) and up to two premature extrastimuli was performed. Premature extrastimuli was decreased in 20 ms step until a coupling interval of 200 ms or the VRP was reached or VF lasting >10 seconds was induced. The induction with PVS up to two premature beats is independent predictors of poor prognosis with a high negative predictive value and was associated with increased risk, but has a controversial prognostic value. The lack of induction does not necessarily portend a low risk and hence clinical factors are the most important determinants [6, 20, 25, 26]. VF inducibility rate is highest in patients with BrS and syncope of unknown origin (80%), the lowest in asymptomatic patients (61.5%), and intermediate in patients with vasovagal syncope (70.5%) [26–29]. However, it is important to note that these observations correspond to the pre-ablation era of BrS and therefore, the PVS could be a good predictor of outcome after RFA [18]. In our patients the endocardial RFA of diastolic electrical activity and abnormal systolic EGMs suppressed the type 1 ECG BrS pattern and inducibility with PVS, making the patients asymptomatic, as was previously reported for the epicardial RFA [17, 18].

We identified three zones of substrate according to amplitude of the systolic EGMs: central very low voltage zone <0.5 mV, peripheral low voltage zone of 0.5–1.5 mV (border) and normal voltage zone >1.5 mV [19]. The central zone of substrate using filling scaling was measured in mm² and located in the RVOT. Areas showing low-amplitude signals were mapped with greater point density. Abnormal endocardial electroanatomic voltage maps, characterized by very low-voltage EGMs with clean diastoles in the central area of substrate were found. Only three patients (23%) during bipolar mapping showed fragmented systolic EGMs of low-voltage (≤ 1.5 mV) with duration greater of 80 ms between central and peripheral zone (border zone) of voltage mapping. As shown in **Figure 3**, only in the peripheral zone of substrate the endocardial diastolic EGMs (mean 6.7 ± 1.4 EGMs in two successive sinus cycles) were present. Overall, the median baseline very low voltage or central area of substrate (≤ 0.5 mV) was 14.2 mm² (SD = 10.5) (**Table 1**).

It is important to note, that epicardial mapping may not recognized a substrate located in the septal zone of RVOT. In addition, during epicardial mapping the interposition of fat tissue between the epicardium and the exploratory catheter could decrease the amplitude of the potentials recorded, giving false areas of low voltage. Our study only inclusion 13 patients and may be considered a small size sample [19]. However, our results are consistent allowing us to reach reliable conclusions. We not performed genetic studies. However, it is unlikely that this could affect our observations because mutations have been described in over 24 genes and BrS-susceptibility genes can only partially explain the clinically diagnosed cases.

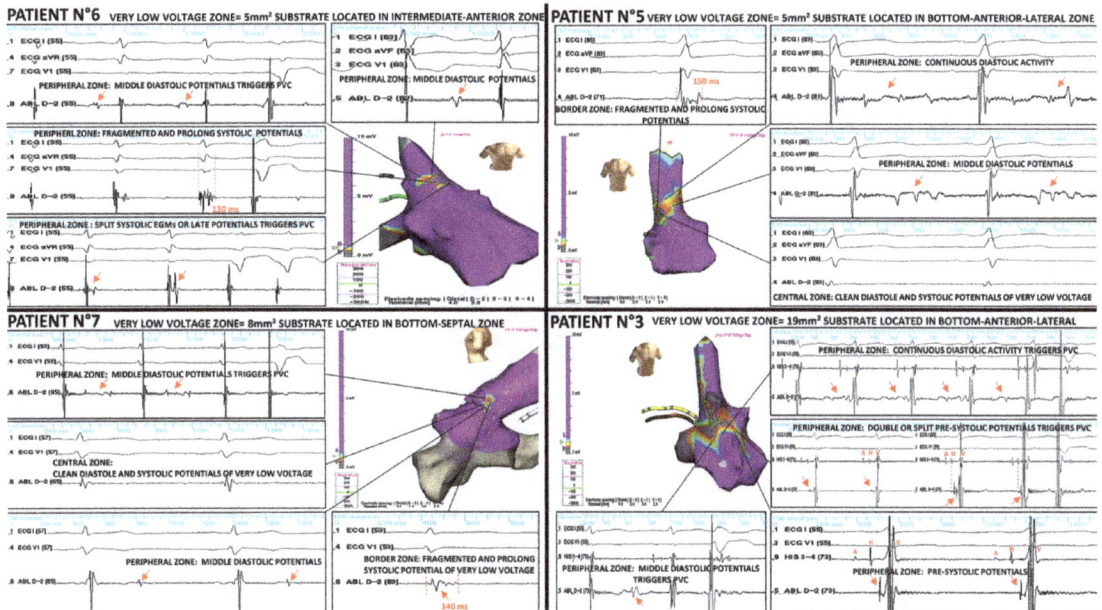

Figure 3. Endocardial electroanatomic maps and location of abnormal EGMs. Double systolic EGMs, late potentials, middle diastolic potentials and continuous diastolic activity in peripheral zone that triggers PVCs is displays. Prolonged and fragmented systolic EGMs of low voltage in border zone in three patients can be observed. In the central zone of substrate observe clean diastole with very low-voltage systolic potentials. The N°3 patient displays single and split pre-systolic potentials in peripheral zone of substrate which triggers PVCs [19].

Patient	1	2	3	4	5	6	7	8	9	10	11	12	13	Total	%	Mean	SD
Age	41	33	57	55	58	27	46	26	24	19	38	38	41			38.7	12.3
Sex	M	F	F	M	F	M	M	F	F	M	F	F	F	F = 8 M = 5	F = 61.5%-M = 38.5%		
Spontaneous type 1 ECG pattern	Yes	Yes	Yes	Yes	Yes	Yes	Yes	Yes	Yes	Yes	Yes	Yes	Yes	13	100%		
Syncope without prodromes	Yes	Yes	Yes	Yes	Yes	Yes	Yes	Yes	Yes	Yes	Yes	Yes	Yes	13	100%		
Nocturnal agonal respiration	No	No	No	No	Yes	No	Yes	No	Yes	No	No	Yes	No	4	31%		
Palpitations	Yes	Yes	Yes	Yes	Yes	Yes	Yes	Yes	Yes	Yes	Yes	Yes	Yes	13	100%		
Family history SCD	No	No	Yes	Yes	Yes	No	No	No	Yes	Yes	Yes	No	No	7	54%		
Family history BrS	No	Yes	No	No	No	No	No	No	Yes	Yes	Yes	No	No	4	31%		
VRP ≤ 200 ms	180	180	160	200	160	180	200	180	160	180	180	200	180	13	100%	180 ms	13.6
QRS duration in V2 lead (> 120 ms)	160	105	120	180	120	120	140	100	90	140	170	140	100	6	46%	129.6 ms	27
R wave in aVR lead (≥ 3 mm) (#)	3	4.5	2	2.5	1.5	1	4	4	1.5	6	3	4	1	7	54%	3 mm	1.4
QRS fragmentation	No	Yes	No	No	No	No	No	Yes	No	No	No	No	Yes	3	23%		
J wave	No	No	No	No	No	Yes	Yes	No	No	No	Yes	No	No	2	15.4%		
HV interval to DI lead (>55 ms)	60	57	40	120	57	40	46	35	45	45	55	35	59	5	38.5%	53.4 ms	21
HV interval to V2 lead (>55 ms)	40	40	35	80	45	40	46	35	40	45	55	35	46	1	7.7%	44.8 ms	11.5
Follow-up (months)	66	63	56	53	51	54	45	46	45	43	28	12	19	13	100%	44.7	15.5
CDI implant	No	Yes	Yes	Yes	Yes	Yes	No	Yes	Yes	Yes	Yes	Yes	No	10	77%		
Biopsy	No	No	No	No	No	Yes	No	No	No	No	Yes	No	Yes	2	15%		
Very low-voltage AREA(≤ 0.5 mV) in (mm²)	23	8	19	42	5	4	8	10	19	10	8	25	4	13	100%	14.2 mm²	10.5
N° endocardial diastolic EGMs IN 2 successive cycles sinus (≥4 EGMs)	8	8	5	7	7	9	6	6	9	6	6	7	4	13	100%	6.7	1.4
Procedure time (min)	120	110	100	90	120	95	105	95	100	100	160	90	170			112	24.5
Fluoroscopy time (min)	15	10	10	10	15	10	12	13	12	10	27	10	25			13.7	5.5

M = male, F = female, SD = standard deviation, (#) = during flecainide test, VRP = ventricular refractory period.
Source: Ref. [19].

Table 1. Basal characteristic and risk factors.

Although the results of mapping and RFA were good, we do not perform epicardial mapping and do not ignore the possibility that a portion of the substrate can remain present after ablation.

In addition, we found pre-systolic potentials as was previously reported by Haissaguerre et al. [15]. We showed with TEM Purkinje fibers in RVOT (**Figures 2** and **3**) [19]. These could be involved in the origin of pre-systolic potentials and genesis of early-onset PVCs that can trigger VT or VF, by spontaneous depolarization or micro-reentry circuit in the Purkinje network [30].

4. Electrocardiographic analysis

4.1. Size of substrate and ST-segment elevation

In the BrS the mechanism of ST segment elevation has been explained by the repolarization theory (decreased of Na + and/or Ca++ channel function with a prominent Ito current in epicardium of RVOT generates a transmural voltage gradient), or the depolarization theory (disturbances in depolarization of RVOT can be cause of delayed conduction and ST segment elevation) [18, 20]. Nevertheless, the ECG changes are actually explained by the theorem of solid angle, where a substrate larger increases the magnitude of the ST segment elevation [31]. In 13 patients of high risk we have analyzed QRS complex duration, R wave amplitude in aVR lead, presence of fragmented QRS (f-QRS) and end-QRS slur or notch in DI, aVL, DII, DIII and aVF leads with J point peak $\geq$0.2 mv with descending ST segment, corresponding to an early repolarization or "J wave" [19]. Before of endocardial mapping the patients were underwent flecainide testing (400 mg, orally) with the purpose of measuring the greatest ST-segment elevation. The partial greatest ST-segment elevation in millimeters (ST-segment elevation in V1 + V2 leads in the third ICS and ST-segment elevation in V1 + V2 + V3 leads in fourth ICS), and total sum of greatest ST-segment elevation (ST segment elevation in V1 + V2 leads in the third ICS plus ST-segment elevation in V1 + V2 + V3 leads in fourth ICS) were measured. (**Figure 4-A**). Correlation between size and location of substrate in the electro-anatomic map and the ST-segment elevation were analyzed. As shown in **Figure 4** and **Table 2**, with a cut-off $\geq$13 mm in the total sum of ST segment elevation two variants were found: (1) A total sum of ST-segment elevation <13 mm (n = 8, 61.5%, mean 9.6 ± 1.3 mm) corresponded to a central area of substrate of 7.7 ± 1.8 mm^2; (2) A total sum of ST segment elevation $\geq$13 mm (n = 5, 38.5%, mean 15 ± 1.1 mm) corresponded to a central area of substrate of 28.2 ± 9.2 mm^2 (p < 0.001 for correlation of ST segment elevation and correlation of central area of substrate, with a value >0.90 of ROC curve).

Brugada et al. during electro-anatomic mapping with administration of a sodium channel blocker showed an increase in the size of the low voltage [18]. In concordance, our observations suggest that the total sum of ST segment elevation during flecainide testing would approximately determine the substrate size. In addition, the ECG leads with greater ST segment elevation would locate the substrate in the RVOT [19].

Morita et al. (145 patients who experienced syncope or had VF events) proposes ECG risk markers for the initial and recurrent episodes of VF in symptomatic patients with BrS. The f-QRS,

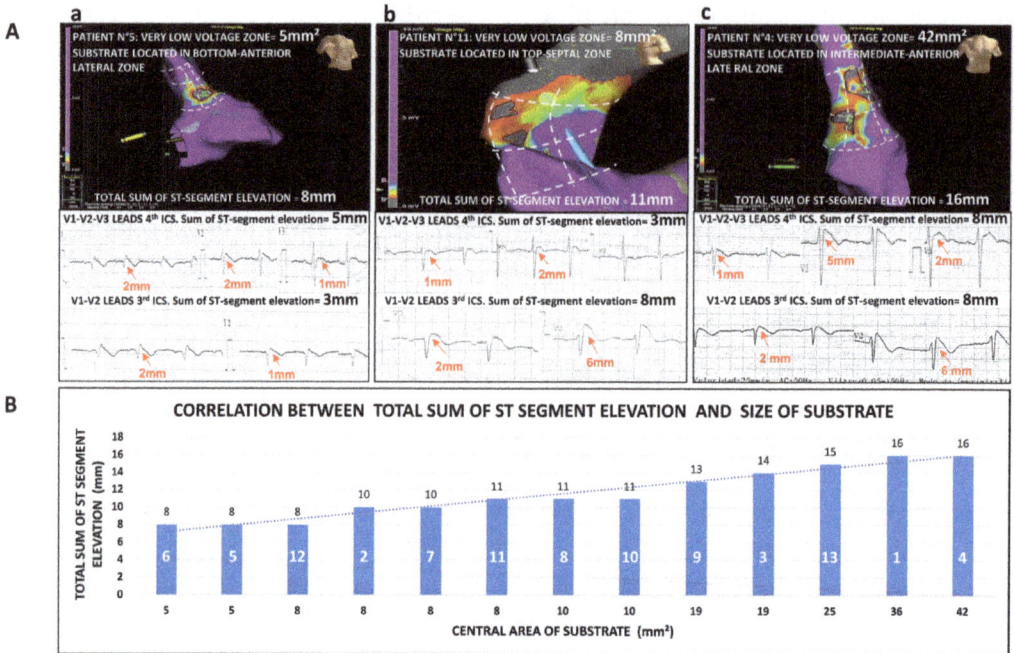

Figure 4. Correlation between ST segment elevation and substrate localization. A. With the administration of sodium channel blocker, a greater magnitude of total sum of ST segment elevation corresponds to a greater very low voltage area of substrate, and allows its location in the longitudinal plane of RVOT. (a) The location of the substrate in the bottom zone of RVOT correspond to a greater sum of ST segment elevation in fourth ICS vs. third ICS (5 vs. 3 mm). (b) The location of the substrate in the top zone of RVOT correspond to a greater sum of ST segment elevation in third ICS vs. 4th ICS (8 vs. 3 mm). (c) The location of the substrate in the intermediate zone of RVOT corresponds to a sum of ST segment elevation of equal magnitude in third ICS and fourth ICS (8 mm and 8 mm). B. The graph shows the correlation between linear increase of total sum of ST segment elevation and substrate size. The blue bars indicate each patient [19].

inferolateral early repolarization and complete RBBB were associated with occurrence of ventricular tachyarrhythmia in the symptomatic patients [34]. Our population show in three patients a QRS fragmentation (23%) and in two patients a J wave (15.4%) [19].

4.2. Location of substrate in the longitudinal plane

Nademanee et al. found functional substrate in the anterior zone of epicardium of RVOT [17]. Brugada et al. in 14 inducible patients reported a functional substrate in epicardium of RVOT and anterior free wall of right ventricle [18].

In our study a high-density endocardial electroanatomical mapping of right ventricle and RVOT was performed [19]. Taking the pulmonary valve as upper limit and the supraventricular crest as lower limit in the longitudinal plane the RVOT was divided in top and bottom. As shown in **Figure 4-A** and Table II, we have found three variants: (1) When the substrate was located in the top region of RVOT, it corresponded with the greater sum of ST-segment elevation in V1-V2 leads in the 3rd ICS (n = 5, 38.5%); (2) When the substrate was located in the bottom region of RVOT (n = 5, 38.5%), it corresponded with the greater sum of ST-segment elevation in V1-V2-V3 leads in the 4th ICS; (3) When the substrate was located in

Patient	ST-segment with	Total sum of ST-segment	Size of low voltage	Location of substrate
	>elevation (mm)	Elevation (mm)	Area (mm²)	In the longitudinal and
	V1-V2 leads V1-V2-V3 leads			**Transverse plane**
	Third ICS 4TH ICS			
	V1 = 2 V1 = 2			
1	V2 = 4 V2 = 7	16	36	Bottom
	V3 = 1			Anterior-lateral
	V1 = 3 V1 = 1			
2	V2 = 4 V2 = 2	10	8	Top
	V3 = 0			Anterior-lateral
	V1 = 2 V1 = 3			
3	V2 = 3 V2 = 5	14	19	Bottom
	V3 = 1			Anterior-lateral
	V1 = 2 V1 = 1			
4	V2 = 6 V2 = 5	16	42	Intermediate
	V3 = 2			Anterior-lateral
	V1 = 2 V1 = 2			
5	V2 = 1 V2 = 2	8	5	Bottom
	V3 = 1			Anterior-lateral
	V1 = 2 V1 = 0			
6	V2 = 2 V2 = 2	8	5	Intermediate
	V3 = 2			Anterior
	V1 = 1 V1 = 1			
7	V2 = 3 V2 = 4	10	8	Bottom
	V3 = 1			Septal
	V1 = 3 V1 = 1			
8	V2 = 5 V2 = 2	11	10	Top
	V3 = 0			Anterior
	V1 = 2 V1 = 3			
9	V2 = 3 V2 = 4	13	19	Bottom
	V3 = 1			Anterior-septal
	V1 = 5 V1 = 1			
10	V2 = 3 V2 = 2	11	10	Top
	V3 = 0			Anterior

Patient	ST-segment with >elevation (mm) V1-V2 leads V1-V2-V3 leads Third ICS 4TH ICS	Total sum of ST-segment Elevation (mm)	Size of low voltage Area (mm^2)	Location of substrate In the longitudinal and Transverse plane
	V1 = 2 V1 = 1			
11	V2 = 6 V2 = 2	11	8	Top
	V3 = 0			Septal
	V1 = 2 V1 = 1			
12	V2 = 3 V2 = 2	8	8	Top
	V3 = 0			Anterior-septal
	V1 = 3 V1 = 3			
13	V2 = 4 V2 = 5	15	25	Intermediate
	V3 = 0			Anterior
Mean and SD	3 ± 1.3 2.3 ± 1.5	<13 (n = 8, 61.5%) 9.6 ± 1.3	7.7 ± 1.8	
		≥13 (n = 5, 38.5%) 15 ± 1.1	28.2 ± 9.2	
p value		<0.001	<0.001	

Source: [19].

Table 2. Correlation between sum of ST-segment elevation, location and size of low voltage area.

the intermediate region of RVOT (n = 3, 23%), the sum of ST-segment elevation was of equal magnitude in the 3rd and 4th ICS (n = 3, 23%).

4.3. Location of substrate in the transverse plane

In our study during endocardial electroanatomical mapping, in the transverse plane an anterior, lateral, posterior and septal areas were identified [19]. During endocardial bipolar mapping, the regional depolarization time (RDT) from the endocardial EGM of right ventricular inflow tract (RVIT) recorder by the catheter located at the site of His, until the beginning of endocardial EGM of RVOT, recorded by the catheter located in the RVOT was measured. A value from 0 to 10 ms was considered normal. Moreover, the trans-mural depolarization time (TDT) of RVOT from the beginning of endocardial EGM of RVOT until the end of QRS complex in V2 lead was measured. The TDT measured at DI was considered as normal value. As shown in **Figure 5**, we have found two variants were found: (1) When the substrate was located in the anterior lateral region of RVOT (n = 5, 38.5%), the HV interval measured to DI lead (mean 70.6 ± 24 ms) was longer than the HV interval to V2 lead (mean 50 ± 15 ms). This was accompanied with widening of the QRS complex in its initial and final parts (widening of QRS left and right) in V1 and V2 lead. We defined this as "mixed delay of depolarization of RVOT".

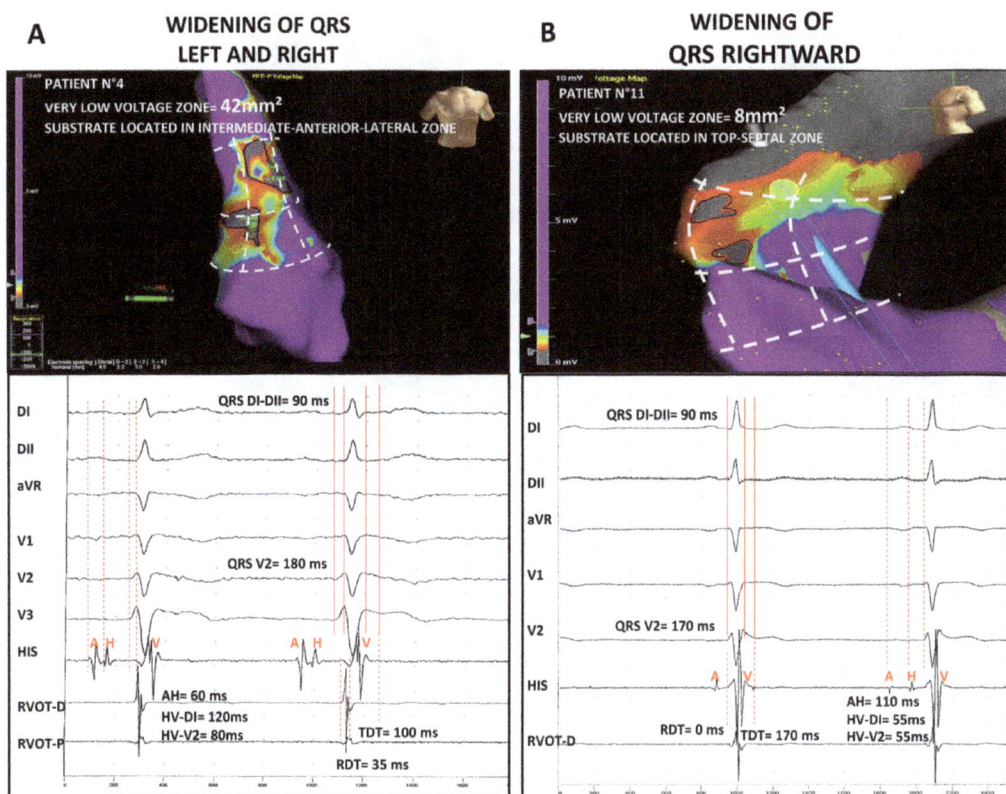

Figure 5. Location of substrate in transverse plane of RVOT. A. The N°4 patient displays a substrate located in the anterior-lateral zone of RVOT which corresponds to a widening of QRS complex to left and right. The HV interval to DI lead is longer (120 ms) that the HV interval to V2 lead (80 ms), while RDT and TDT are prolonged. B. The N°11 patient displays a substrate located in the septal zone of RVOT which correspond only to a widening of end QRS complex. The HV interval to DI and V2 leads is equal (55 ms) and only TDT is prolonged [19].

Simultaneously, TDT and RDT were prolonged, because early depolarization of RVOT occurs. (2) When the substrate was located only in the anterior part (30.8%), or anterior-septal (15.4%) or exclusively in the septal region (15.4%) of RVOT, the HV interval measured to DI and V2 leads showed no increase in its duration (mean 42.6 ± 6 ms and 41 ± 6.5 ms, respectively) and the widening of QRS was only rightward (widening QRS rightward). Moreover, the endocardial EGM of RVIT and RVOT, and beginning of QRS complex in DI-V1-V2 lead they were activated simultaneously, indicating that there is no RDT delay, while TDT of RVOT was prolonged of dynamic manner. We defined this as "end delay depolarization of RVOT".

Was report that 11% of patients with BrS have early repolarization pattern in the inferior-lateral leads and a more severe phenotype [32]. Interestingly, as shown in **Figure 6** we found in two patients who had a substrate of exclusively septal location, showed end-QRS notching or slurring pattern. When the substrate was located in the bottom-septal zone of RVOT (patient N°7) only end-QRS notch in aVL lead and slurred S-wave in DII, DIII and a VF leads was observed (**Figure 6-A**). Whereas, when the substrate was located in the top-septal zone of RVOT (patient N°11) an end-QRS slur in DI and aVL leads was observed (**Figure 6-B**). Our observations suggest that a location of substrate in septal region of RVOT, with beginning of the depolarization at the

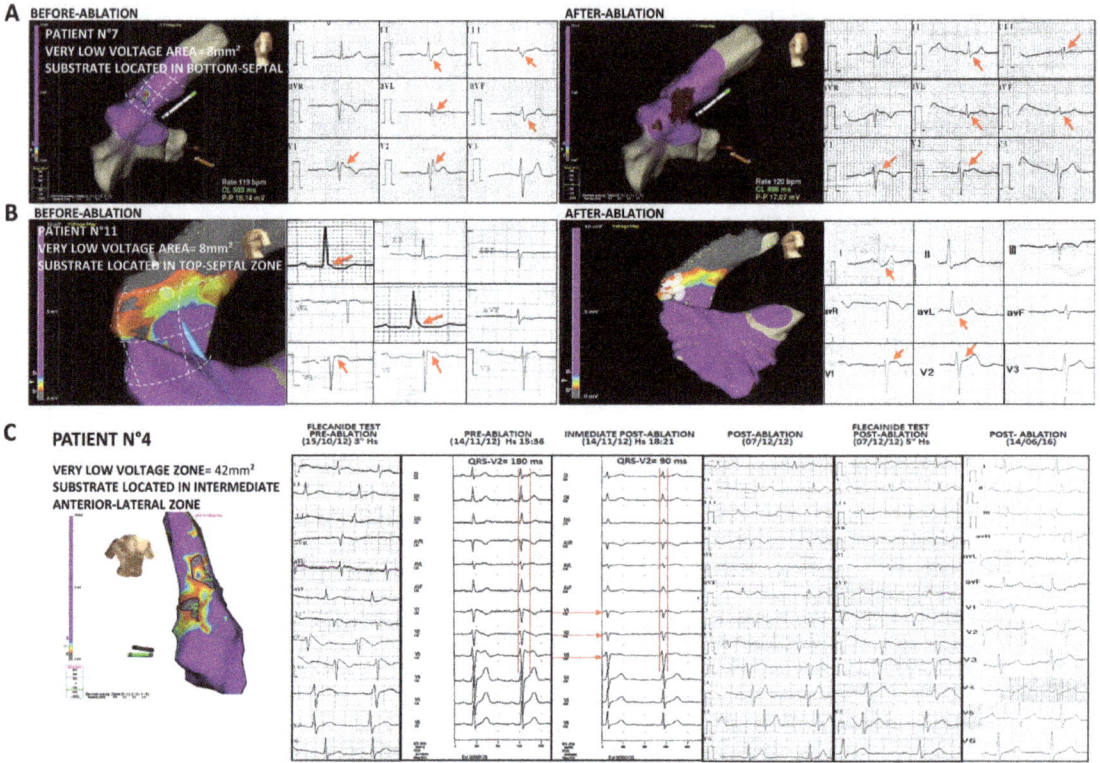

Figure 6. RFA effects on the ECG. A. The N°7 patient displays a substrate located in bottom septal zone of RVOT. Before RFA a type 2 ECG BrS pattern, end-QRS notch in aVL lead and slurred S wave in DII, DIII and aVF leads are present. It disappears after RFA (red arrows). B. The N°11 patient displays a substrate in the top septal zone of RVOT. Before RFA a type 1 ECG BrS pattern and end-QRS slur in DI and aVL leads are present. It disappears after RFA (red arrows). C. Before RFA the flecainide test showed a type 1 ECG BrS pattern. The QRS complex duration in V1 and V2 leads was 180 ms, while in DI was 90 ms (red lines). Immediately after ablation, the duration of QRS complex in V2 lead decreased to 90 ms and ECG BrS pattern disappears (red arrows). After RFA the flecainide test not induced type 1 ECG BrS pattern. The ECG at 3.8 years follow-up persist normal [19].

endocardium correlated with the presence of end-QRS notching or slurring pattern in inferior or/and lateral leads by slow conduction. As shown in **Figure 6 A** and **B** the endocardial RFA of substrate produced their disappearance [19]. Normally the epicardium is electropositive with respect to electronegative endocardium creating a current flow of endocardium to epicardium. When activation spreads from endocardium to epicardium, in a context of slow conduction, the J wave coincides with the notch in the epicardial AP mediated by the Ito current and it is recorded by ECG. Conversely, when the activation begins in the epicardium, the J wave disappears hidden by the QRS complex [33]. Consequently, our observations lead us to think that the J wave depends more of late depolarization that early repolarization as was suggested by other authors.

5. Effects of RFA on the ECG BrS pattern and substrate

Endocardial and epicardial RFA has been proposed as a new strategy to prevent SCD and VT/VF in BrS patients of high risk. Nademanee et al. found what RFA on prolonged and fractionated late potentials in the anterior zone of epicardium of RVOT normalized the ECG BrS pattern and prevented VT/VF in all but one patient during a follow-up of 20 ± 6 months [17]. Recently, Brugada et al. in 14 inducible patients reported abnormal EGMs only in epicardium of the anterior free wall of right ventricle and in RVOT. RFA eliminated both ECG BrS pattern and inducibility, with a median follow-up of 5 months [18].

In our study, the endocardial RFA in 13 patients resulted in normalization of the ECG BrS pattern, disappearance of end-QRS notching or slurring and suppression of inducibility in all patients during a mean follow-up of 47.7 ± 15.5 months (**Table 1**) [19]. About 30 days after RFA a flecainide testing did not develop ECG BrS pattern. Seven patients who entered to procedure with spontaneous type 1 ECG pattern showed ECG normalization at the end of the procedure. Immediately after RFA was applied, activity and varying degrees of changes in ST segment were observed. With following applications of RFA the ECG pattern progressively decreased (**Figure 7**). After RFA local abnormal diastolic EGMs completely disappear and systolic EGMs were replaced by residual very low voltage areas. The mean time of procedure and fluoroscopy were 112 ± 24.5 and 13.7 ± 5.5 minutes, respectively (Table I). Postprocedure, predischarge, and follow-up 12-lead ECG confirmed the absence of BrS ECG pattern (**Figure 6C**). The patients were asymptomatic and free of arrhythmic events in the 24-hour ambulatory ECG monitoring and in follow-up the ICD interrogation. Two patients (15%) had a near-syncope with prodrome at 24 of 46 months and at 18 of 36 months of follow-up respectively, without arrhythmias in ICD interrogation.

Sunsaneewitayakul et al. reported that endocardial RFA on the late depolarization zones modified the ECG BrS pattern in three patients and suppress the VF storm in four patients, during follow-up of 12–30 months [16]. Similarly, we obtained suppression of inducibility, normalization of BrS ECG pattern and early repolarization pattern with endocardial RFA of

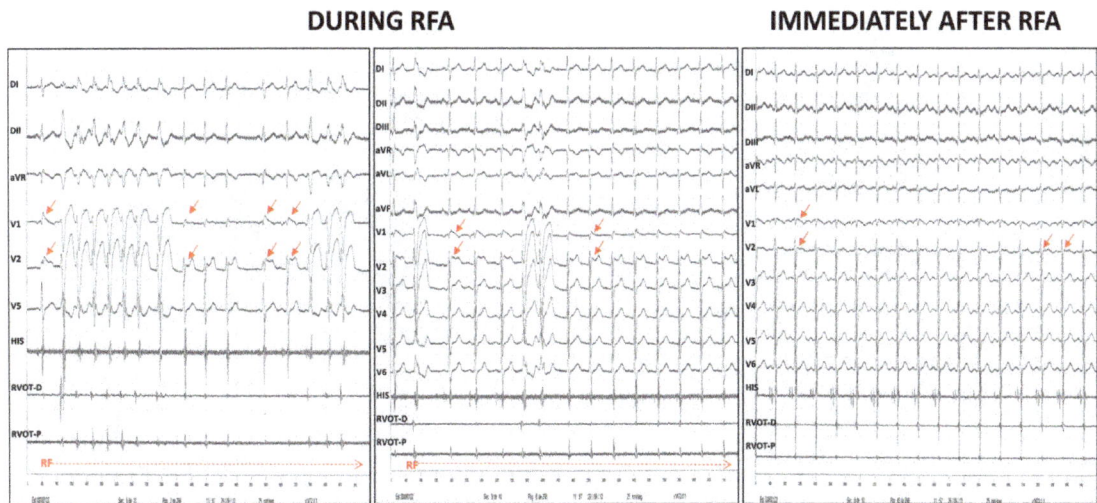

DURING RFA   **IMMEDIATELY AFTER RFA**

Figure 7. Effects of radiofrequency ablation on ECG. In the N°3 patient during endocardial RFA, intense activity and varying degrees of ST segment changes are shown. The ECG pattern progressively decreases with the following applications (red arrows). After RFA the local abnormal diastolic EGMs completely disappeared and systolic EGMs were replaced by residual low voltage areas [19].

areas with late depolarization, diastolic electrical activity and abnormal systolic EGMs [19]; probably by substrate homogenization and transmural lesion of the thin wall of RVOT (mean 3 mm). In addition, as show **Figures 2** and **3** we found pre-systolic potentials as was previously reported by Haissaguerre et al. [15]. In our patients the endocardial RFA of these potentials suppress PVCs and inducibility on PVS [19].

6. Correlation between functional and ultrastructural substrate

Coronel et al. show in a heart explanted of a BrS patient, fibrosis with epicardial fat infiltration as well as conduction slow without transmural repolarization differences [35]. Furthermore, interstitial fibrosis, fat tissue and myocyte disorganization with reduced gap junction expression in the presence of fractionated and unfractionated low voltage systolic EGMs in the endocardium and epicardium of RVOT was reported with optical microscopy [36–38].

In two patients, before RFA and after right internal jugular venous access through a steerable sheath we advanced a bioptome to RVOT and connected to 3-dimensional (3D) mapping system [19]. Guiding by electroanatomic and voltage map two samples of endo-myocardial biopsies of the three previously defined zones of substrate was obtained. Samples were fixed in 4% glutaraldehyde and 0.1% sodium phosphate (pH 7.4) for transmission electron microscopy (TEM) study as was described previously [39]. As show **Figure 8** the ultrastructural substrate and functional substrate were correlated [19]. In the **Figure 8A**, the patient N°13 in (a), (d) and (g) shows electro-anatomic and voltage map (functional substrate) with a central area of substrate of 25 mm^2 located in the intermediate-anterior zone of the RVOT and the bioptome

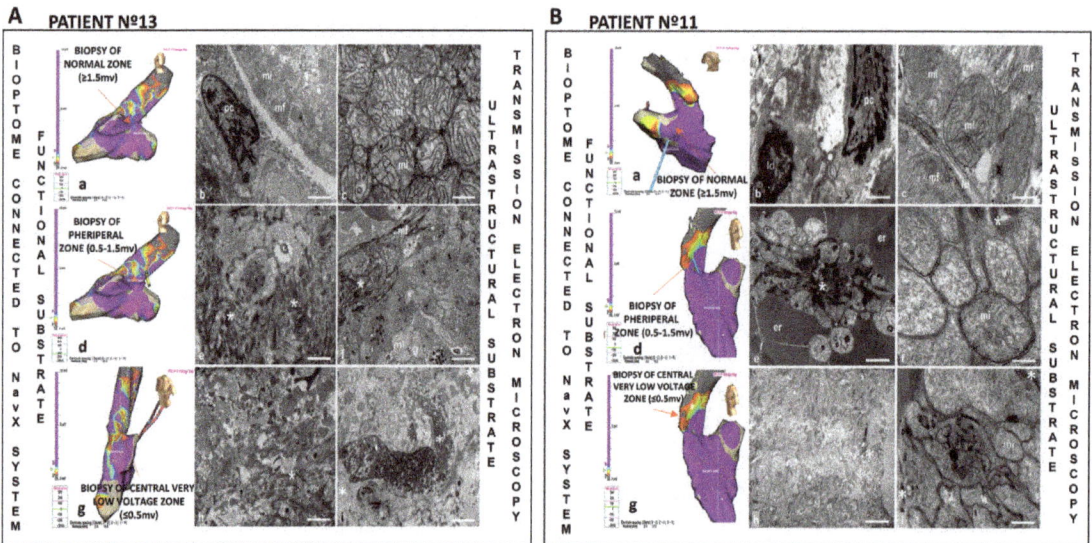

Figure 8. Correlation between functional and ultrastructural substrate. On the left side the electro-anatomic and voltage map (functional substrate) and bioptome connected to the navigation system is shown. On the right side the ultrastructural substrate is shown. Scale Barr: 3.33, 2.2 and 1.42 μm; mitochondria (mi); myofibrils (mf); Purkinje cell (pc); myofibrillar rests (*); lipofusin deposit (ld); intercalated disk (id); remains of erythrocytes (er) [19].

connected to the navigation system. In (b) and (c) on the right side can be seen the ultra-structural substrate which corresponds to normal zone with mitochondria, myofibrils, and a Purkinje cell of normal characteristics. In contrast, in the peripheral zone of substrate (e and f) note that when approaching to pathological area, cytoplasmic vacuolization, myofibrillar and mitochondrial disorganization with myofibrillar residue can be observed. The (h) and (i) corresponds to the central zone, which depicts strong vacuolization and cell destruction with intense cytoplasmic disorganization and myofibrillar residue. In the **Figure 8B**, the patient N° 11 in (a), (d) and (g) shows the voltage and electro-anatomic map (functional substrate) with central area of substrate of 8mm² located in the top-septal zone of the RVOT. In (b) and (c) on the right side can be seen the ultrastructural substrate which corresponds to normal zone with normal characteristics of mitochondria, myofibrils, and a Purkinje cell. The approaching to pathologi-cal area in the peripheral zone of substrate (e and f), myofibrillar disorganization, citoplas-mic vacuolization, swelling and disappearance of mitochondrial crests, myofibrillar rests and remains of erythrocytes were observed. The (h) and (i) corresponds to the central zone showing strong vacuolization and cell destruction and myofibrillar residue. Fat replacement, lympho-cytic infiltration, Chagasic myocarditis, collagen tissue or apoptotic bodies were not observed.

It is important to note that when we approach to pathological areas progressive cell damage was observed. In the central zone of substrate low voltage systolic EGMs coincided with strong cell destruction and cytoplasmic disorganization. The peripheral zone of substrate with cell damage, mitochondrial swelling and myofibrillar residue without apoptotic bodies coincided with late potentials, diastolic and/or presystolic activity (**Figures 2** and **3**). These findings support mitochondrial energy loss as possible non-apoptotic progressive tissue damage and death cell. Our results suggest the interesting possibility that substrate could be generated by an abnormal expression of neural crest cells localized in RVOT during cardiac development. Because an epicardial and endocardial substrate was demonstrated, our findings together with those of other researchers support the probability of a transmural substrate.

7. Mechanisms of arrhythmias

Two theories suggest that an abnormal repolarization (local re-excitation by phase 2 reentry in the epicardium) or a defect of the depolarization (disturbances in depolarization of RVOT can cause conduction delay) may be responsible of phenotype and VF in BrS [40–43]. However, in BrS the arrhythmias are usually polymorphic VT or VF, and these cannot be supported by macro-reentry mechanisms. VF depends of a firing focus initiated by early or delayed after-depolarization or a micro-re-entry [44]. Surviving cells surrounded by fibrosis has demon-strated to be responsible of slow conduction and reentry in inhomogeneous scars [45]. The residual electrical activity within scar was reported as delayed or isolated EGMs, late potentials or diastolic EGMs and their elimination during sinus rhythm was effective to prevent VT/VF [45]. In peripheral zone of substrate when a sufficient degree of cell damage was reached such as we found with TEM and resting potentials are reduced the polymorphic VT/VF may occur. This event could be originated through a firing focus or by multiple wavelets from a reentrant microcircuit, and would explain the "diastolic electrical activity" observed in our patients.

In addition, we found pre-systolic potentials as was previously reported by Haissaguerre et al. [15]. As show **Figure 8**, the Purkinje fibers in RVOT could be involved in the origin of pre-systolic potentials and in genesis of early-onset PVCs that can trigger VT or VF, by spontaneous depolarization or micro-reentry circuit in the Purkinje network [30].

8. Conclusion

In patients with BrS of high risk the substrate RFA may be a potential option of treatment. We successfully ablated the substrate of BrS from the endocardium based on the electrophysiological and ultrastructural findings. Our data together with the observations of other researchers suggest a transmural substrate, contributing to future definition of the arrhythmogenic substrate in BrS. As many phenotypes are involved in BrS, it is not unthinkable that different substrates may exist in BrS. ECG analysis during administration of a sodium channel blocker allows approximately determined the size and location of substrate. Careful endocardial mapping allows identify late potentials, presystolic and diastolic EGMs as a new risk marker to guide an endocardial substrate RFA, probably with the same results what a more complex epicardial ablation. A comparative study between endocardial and epicardial RFA should be performed.

Acknowledgements

This research was supported by funding sources from the Electrophysiology Division (Model Heart Center) to PET, and PIP 2015 No.183 (CONICET Argentina) and PICT 2013 No. 1949 (ANPCyT, Argentina) grants to SSS and SMH. We thank to Abbott-Argentina for providing financial support to publication.

Conflict of interest

The authors declare none conflict of interest.

Abbreviations

AP	action potential
BrS	Brugada syndrome
ECG	electrocardiogram
EGMs	electrograms
EPS	electrophysiology study
f-QRS	fragmented QRS

ICD	implantable cardioverter defibrillator
LPs	late potentials
PVC	premature ventricular contractions
PVS	programmed ventricular stimulation
RFA	radiofrequency ablation
RP	refractory period
RV	right ventricle
RVIT	right ventricular inflow tract
RVOT	right ventricular outflow tract
SCD	sudden cardiac death
TEM	transmission electron microscopy
VF	ventricular fibrillation
VRP	ventricular refractory period
VT	ventricular tachycardia

Author details

Pablo E. Tauber[1,2]*, Virginia Mansilla[1], Pedro Brugada[3], Sara S. Sánchez[4], Stella M. Honoré[4], Marcelo Elizari[5], Sergio Chain Molina[1], Felix A. Albano[2], Ricardo R. Corbalán[1], Federico Figueroa Castellanos[6] and Damian Alzugaray Bioeng[7]

*Address all correspondence to: pablotauber@gmail.com

1 Model Heart Center, Electrophysiology Division, Laprida, San Miguel de Tucumán, Argentina

2 ZJS Hospital Health Center, Unit of Arrhythmias and Electrophysiology, San Miguel de Tucumán, Argentina

3 Cardiovascular Institute, Cardiovascular Division, Free University of Brussels, UZ Brussel-VUB, Brussels, Belgium

4 Department of Developmental Biology, INSIBIO (National Council for Scientific and Technical Research-National University of Tucumán), Chacabuco, San Miguel de Tucumán, Argentina

5 Emeritus FACC, National Academy of Medicine, Buenos Aires, Argentina

6 Clinica Mayo de UMCB, Unit of Arrhythmias and Electrophysiology, San Miguel de Tucumán, Argentina

7 Abbott, Argentina

References

[1] Brugada P, Brugada J. Right bundle branch block, persistent ST segment elevation and sudden cardiac death: A distinct clinical and electrocardiographic syndrome: A multi-center report. Journal of the American College of Cardiology. 1992;**20**:1391-1396

[2] Postema PG, van Dessel PF, de Bakker JMT, Dekker LRC, Linnenbank AC, Hoogendijk MG, Coronel R, Tijssen JGP, Wiildeaam, Tan HL. Slow and discontinuous conduction conspire in Brugada syndrome: A right ventricular mapping and stimulation study. Cir culation: Arrhythmia and Electrophysiology. 2008;**1**:7379-7386

[3] Nagase S, Kusano KF, Morita H, Fujimoto Y, Kakishita M, Nakamura K, Emori T, Matsubara H, Ohe T. Epicardial electrogram of the right ventricular outflow tract in patients with the Brugada syndrome: Using the epicardial lead. Journal of the American College of Cardiology. 2002;**39**:1992-1995

[4] Elizari MV, Levi R, Acunzo RS, Chiale PA, Civetta MM, Ferreiro M, Sicouri S. Abnormal expression of cardiac neural crest cells in heart development: A different hypothesis for the etiopathogenesis of Brugada syndrome. Heart Rhythm. 2007;**4**:359-365

[5] Bayés De Luna A, Brugada P, Baranchuk A, Borggrefe M, Breithardt G, Goldwasser LP, Pérez Riera A, Garcia-Niebla J, Pastore C, Oreto G, McKenna W, Zareba W, Brugada R, Brugada P. Current electrocardiographic criteria for diagnosis of Brugada pattern: A consensus report. Journal of Electrocardiology. 2012;**45**:433-442

[6] Delise P, Allocca G, Sitta N. Risk of sudden death in subjects with Brugada type 1 electrocardiographic pattern and no previous cardiac arrest: Is it high enough to justify an extensive use of prophylactic ICD? Journal of Cardiovascular Medicine (Hagerstown, Md.) 2016;**17**:408-410. PMID: 27116235. DOI: 10.2459/JCM.0000000000000253

[7] Priori SG, Blomstrom-Lundqvist C, Mazzanti A, et al. 2015 ESC guidelines for the management of patients with ventricular arrhythmias and the prevention of sudden cardiac death: The Task Force for the Management of Patients with Ventricular Arrhythmias and the Prevention of Sudden Cardiac Death of the European Society of Cardiology (ESC). Endorsed by: Association for European Paediatric and Congenital Cardiology (AEPC). European Heart Journal. 2015;**36**:2793-2867

[8] Bonny A, Talle MA, Vaugrenard T, Taieb J, Ngantcha M. Inappropriate implantable cardioverter defibrillator shocks in Brugada syndrome: Pattern in primary and secondary prevention. Indian Pacing and Electrophysiology Journal. 2017;**17**:10-15

[9] Priori SG, Wilde AA, Horie M, Cho Y, Behr ER, Berul C, Nico Blom N, Brugada J, Chiang C, HuikuriH, Kannankeril P, Krahn A, Leenhardt A, Moss A, Schwartz PJ, Shimizu W, Tomaselli G, Tracy C. Executive summary: HRS/EHRA/APHRS expert consensus statement on the diagnosis and management of patients with inherited primary arrhythmia syndromes. Europace. 2013;**15**:1389-1406

[10] Kapplinger JD, Tester DJ, Alders M, Benito B, Berthet M, Brugada J, Brugada P, Fressart V, Guerchicoff A, Harris-Kerr C, Kamakura S, Kyndt F, Koopmann T, Miyamoto Y,

Pfeiffer R, Pollevick G, Probst V, Zumhagen S, Vatta M, Towbin J, Shimizu W, Schulze-Bahr E, Antzelevitch C, Salisbury B, Guicheney P, Wilde A, Ramon Brugada R, Schott J-J, Ackerman M. An international compendium of mutations in the SCN5A-encoded cardiac sodium channel in patients referred for Brugada syndrome genetic testing. Heart Rhythm. 2010;**7**:33-46

[11] Fernandez-Falgueras A, Sarquella-Brugada G, Brugada J, Brugada R, Campuzano O. Cardiac channelopathies and sudden death: Recent clinical and genetic advances. Biology (Basel). 2017;**6**(1):1-21

[12] Sacher F, Jesel L, Jais P, Haïssaguerre M. Insight into the mechanism of Brugada syndrome: Epicardial substrate and modification during ajmaline testing. Heart Rhythm. 2014;**11**:732-734. DOI: 10.1016/j. hrthm.2013.05.023

[13] Tauber PE, Mansilla V, Mercau G, Albano F, Corbalán RR, Sánchez SS, Honoré SM. Correlation between functional and ultrastructural substrate in Brugada syndrome. Heart Rhythm Case Reports. 2016;**2**(3):211-216

[14] Kofune M, Watanabe I, Ohkubo K, Ashino S, Okumura Y, Nagashima K, Mano H, Nakai T, Kasamaki Y, Hirayama A. Clarifying the arrhythmogenic substrate for Brugada syndrome. Electroantomic mapping study of the right ventricle. International Heart Journal. 2011;**52**:290-294

[15] Haissaguerre M, Extramiana F, Hocini M, Cauchemez B, Jais P, Cabrera J, Farre G, Leenhardt A, Sanders P, Scavee C, Hsu LF, Weerasooriya R, Shah D, Frank R, Maury P, Garrigue S, Clementy J. Mapping and ablation of ventricular fibrillation associated with long-QT and Brugada syndromes. Circulation. 2003;**108**:925-928

[16] Sunsaneewitayakul B, Yao Y, Thamaree S, Zhang S. Endocardial mapping and catheter ablation for ventricular fibrillation prevention in Brugada syndrome. Journal of Cardiovascular Electrophysiology. 2012;**23**(Sup. s1):1-7

[17] Nademanee K, Veerakul G, Chandanamattha P, Chaothawee L, Ariyachaipanich A, Jirasirirojanakorn K, Likittanasombat K, Bhuripanyo K, Ngarmukos T. Prevention of ventricular fibrillation episodes in Brugada syndrome by catheter ablation over the anterior right ventricular outflow tract Epicardium. Circulation. 2011;**123**:1270-1279

[18] Brugada J, Pappone C, Berruezo A, Vicedomini G, Manguso F, Ciconte G, Giannelli L, Santinelli V. Brugada syndrome phenotype elimination by epicardial substrate ablation. Circulation. Arrhythmia and Electrophysiology. 2015;**8**:1373-1381

[19] Tauber P, MansillaV, Brugada P, Sánchez S, Honoré SM, Elizari M, Molina S, Albano FA, Corbalán R, Figueroa Castellanos F, Alzugaray D. Endocardial approach for substrate ablation in brugada syndrome: Epicardial, endocardial or transmural substrate? Journal of Clinical and Experimental Research in Cardiology. 2018;**4**(1). ISSN: 2394-6504 (in press)

[20] Sieira J, Conte G, Ciconte G, Chierchia GB, Casado-Arroyo R, Baltogiannis G, Di Giovanni G, Saitoh Y, Juliá J, Mugnai G, La Meir M, Wellens F, Czapla J, Pappaert G,

de Asmundis C, Brugada P. A score model to predict risk of events in patients with Brugada syndrome. European Heart Journal. 2017;**38**:1756-1763

[21] Nakazawa K, Tsuneharu Sakurai T, Takagi A, Kishi R, Osada K, Nanke T, Miyake F, Matsumoto N, Kobayashi S. Autonomic imbalance as a property of symptomatic Brugada syndrome. Circulation Journal. 2003;**67**:511-514

[22] Mizumaki K, Fujiki A, Tsuneda T, Sakabe M, Nishida K, Sugao M, Inoue H. Vagal activity modulates spontaneous augmentation of ST elevation in the daily life of patients with Brugada syndrome. Journal of Cardiovascular Electrophysiology. 2004 Jun;**15**(6):667-673

[23] Alboni P, Brignole M, Menozzi C, Raviele A, Del Rosso A, Dinelli M, Solano A, Bottoni N. Diagnostic value of history in patients with syncope with or without heart disease. Journal of the American College of Cardiology. 2001 Jun 1;**37**(7):1921-1928

[24] Shimizu W, Matsuo K, Kokubo Y, et al. Sex hormone and gender difference: Role of testosterone on male predominance in Brugada syndrome. Journal of Cardiovascular Electrophysiology. 2007;**18**:415-421

[25] Delise P, Allocca G, Sitta N. Brugada type 1 electrocardiogram: Should we treat the electrocardiogram or the patient? World Journal of Cardiology. 2017 September 26;**9**(9):737-741

[26] Sroubek J, Probst V, Mazzanti A, Delise P, Castro Hevia J, Ohkubo K, Zorzi A, Champagne J, Kostopoulou A, Yin X, Napolitano C, Milan DJ, Wilde A, Sacher F, Borggrefe M, Ellinor PT, Theodorakis G, Nault I, Corrado D, Watanabe I, Antzelevitch C, Allocca G, Priori SG, Lubitz SA. Programmed ventricular stimulation for risk stratification in the brugada syndrome. A pooled analysis. Circulation. 2016;**133**:622-630

[27] Belhassen B, Rahkovich M, Michowitz Y, Glick A, Viskin S. Management of Brugada syndrome thirty-three–year experience using electrophysiologically guided therapy with class 1A antiarrhythmic. Drugs. Circulation: Arrhythmia and Electrophysiology. 2015;**8**:1393-1402. DOI: 10.1161/CIRCEP.115.003109

[28] Sieira J, Conte G, Ciconte G, Carlo de Asmundis, Chierchia G-B, Baltogiannis G, Di Giovanni G, Saitoh Y, Irfan G, Casado-Arroyo R; Juliá J, La Meir M, Wellens F, Wauters K, Van Malderen S, Pappaert G, Brugada P. Prognostic value of programmed electrical stimulation in Brugada syndrome. 20 years' experience. Circulation. Arrhythmia and Electrophysiology 2015;**8**:777-784

[29] Brugada J, Brugada R, Brugada P. Electrophysiologic testing predicts events in Brugada syndrome patients. Heart Rhythm. 2011;**8**:1595-1597

[30] Boyden PA, Dun W, Robins RB. Cardiac Purkinje fibers and arrhythmia; the GK Moe award lecture 2015. Heart Rhythm. 2016;**13**(5):1172-1181

[31] Holland RP, Arnsdorf MF. Solid angle theory and the electrocardiogram: Physiologic and quantitative interpretations. Progress in Cardiovascular Diseases. 1977 May-Jun; **19**(6):431-457

[32] Sarkozy A, Chierchia GB, Paparella G, Boussy T, De Asmundis C, Roos M, Henkens S, Kaufman L, Buyl R, Brugada R, Brugada J, Brugada P. Inferior and lateral electrocardiographic repolarization abnormalities in Brugada syndrome. Circulation. Arrhythmia and Electrophysiology. 2009;**2**:154-161

[33] Postema P, Wilde A. Do J waves constitute a syndrome? Journal of Electrocardiology. 2013;**46**(5):461-465

[34] Morita H, Watanabe A, Satoshi Kawada S, Miyamoto M, Morimoto Y, Nakagawa K, Nishii N, Nakamura K, Ito H. Identification of electrocardiographic risk markers for theinitial and recurrent episodes of ventricular fibrillation inpatients with Brugada syndrome. Journal of Cardiovascular Electrophysiology. 2018;**29**:107-114

[35] Coronel R, Casini S, Koopmann TT, Wilms-Schopman FJG, Verkerk AO, de Groot JR, Bhuiyan Z, Bezzina CR, Veldkamp MW, LinnenbankAC, van der Wal AC, MD, TanHL, MD, Brugada P, MD, Wilde AAM, de Bakker JMT. Right ventricular fibrosis and conduction delay in a patient with clinical signs of Brugada syndrome a combined electrophysiological, genetic, histopathologic, and computational study. Circulation 2005; **112**:2769-2777

[36] Nademanee K, Raju H, Noronha S, Papadakis M, Robinson L, Rothery S, Makita N, Kowase S, Boonmme N, Vitayakritsirikul V, Ratanarapee S, Sharma S, ac V d W, Christiansen M, Tan HL, Wilde A, Nogami A, Sheppard MN, Verakul G, Behr E. Fibrosis, connexin-43, and conduction abnormalities in the Brugada syndrome. Journal of the American College of Cardiology. 2015;**66**:1976-1986

[37] Frustaci A, Priori SG, Pieroni M, Chimenti C, Napolitano C, Rivolta I, Sanna T, Bellocci F, Russo MA. Cardiac histological substrate in patients with clinical phenotype of Brugada syndrome. Circulation. 2005;**112**:3680-3687

[38] Ohkubo K, Watanabe I, Okumura Y, Takagi Y, Ashino S, Kofune M, Sigimura H, Nakai T, Kasamaki Y, Hirayama A, Morimoto SI. Right ventricular histological substrate and conduction delay in patients with Brugada syndrome. International Heart Journal. 2010; **51**:17-23

[39] Sánchez SS, Genta SB, Aybar MJ, Honoré SM, Villecco EI, Sánchez Riera AN. Changes in the expression of small intestine extracellular matrix proteins in streptozotocin-induced diabetic rats. Cell Biology International. 2000;**24**(12):881-888

[40] Antzelevitch C, Fish J, Di Diego JM. Cellular mechanisms underlying the Brugada syndrome. In: Antzelevitch C, Brugada P, Brugada J, Brugada R, editors. The Brugada Syndrome: From Bench to Bedside. Oxford: Blackwell Futura; 2004. pp. 52-77

[41] Postema PG, van Dessel PF, Kors JA, Linnenbank AC, van Herpen G, Ritsema van Eck HJ, van Geloven N, de Bakker J, Wilde A, Tan H. Local depolarization abnormalities are the dominant pathophysiologic mechanism for type 1 electrocardiogram in Brugada syndrome: A study of electrocardiograms, vectorcardiograms, and body surface potential maps during ajmaline provocation. Journal of the American College of Cardiology. 2010;**55**:789-797

[42] Wilde AA, Postema PG, Di Diego JM, Viskin S, Morita H, Fish JM, et al. The pathophysi-
      ological mechanism underlying Brugada syndrome: Depolarization versus repolariza-
      tion. Journal of Molecular and Cellular Cardiology. 2010;**49**:543-553

[43] Martini B, Nava A, Thiene G, Buja GF, Canciani B, Scognamiglio R, Daliento L, Dalla
      Volta S. Ventricular fibrillation without apparent heart disease: Description of six cases.
      American Heart Journal. 1989;**118**:1203-1209. DOI: 10.1016/0002-8703(89)90011-2

[44] Pachón Iglesias M, Jalife J. New concepts on the mechanisms of ventricular fibrillation.
      Revista Española de Cardiología. 2001;**54**:373-382

[45] Jais P, Maury P, Khairy P, Sacher F, Nault I, Komatsu Y, Hocini M, Forclaz A, Jadidi
      A, Weerasooryia R, Shah A, Derval N, Cochet H, Knecht S, Miyazaki S, Nick Linton N,
      Rivard L, Wright M, Wilton S, Scherr D, Pascale P, Roten L, Pederson M, Bordachar P,
      Laurent F, Kim S, Ritter P, Clementy J, Haissaguerre M. Elimination of local abnormal
      ventricular activities. A new end point for substrate modification in patients with scar-
      related ventricular tachycardia. Circulation. 2012;**125**:2184-2196

Atrial Flutter: Diagnosis and Management Strategies

Hamid Reza Bonakdar

Abstract

Atrial flutter (AFL) is a regular, macro reentrant arrhythmia traditionally defined as a supraventricular tachycardia with an atrial rate of 240–320 beats per minute (bpm). Pathophysiology of atrial flutter and atrial fibrillation (AF) is closely related to the similar risk of stroke and they coexist clinically. Atrial flutter is classified to cavotricuspid isthmus (CTI) dependent (or typical) and non-isthmus dependent (atypical). Isthmus is a distinct structure in the right atrium (RA) through which atrial flutter passes and makes a good target for ablation therapy. Ablation is the primary therapy in atrial flutter, particularly in CTI dependent group, with regard to its safety profile and high success rate of approximately 90%. Three-dimensional electroanatomic mapping is progressively being used to ablate atypical forms of atrial flutter.

Keywords: typical flutter, atypical flutter, cavotricuspid isthmus, mapping, isthmus block, differential pacing, entrainment, ablation

1. Introduction

Atrial flutter is between three important atrial arrhythmias resulting remarkable morbidities including heart failure and stroke. Atrial flutter has been defined as a macro-reentrant arrhythmia around an anatomic obstacle with an area larger than 2 cm^2. Fast atrial activation inside the atria produces sinusoidal flutter waves at a rate of 240–320 bpm with no baseline isoelectric, most clearly visible in inferior and V1 leads in the surface ECG. Atrial flutter and fibrillation frequently coexist and atrial flutter can degenerate into atrial fibrillation. With regard to the mechanism of flutter (reentry), this atrial tachyarrhythmia is very amenable to Radiofrequency Ablation (RFA). In this chapter, clinical aspects of atrial flutter will be discussed in detail which includes classification, clinical manifestation, ECG and electrophysiological characteristics and medical or invasive management.

2. Epidemiology

Overall, the incidence of AFL in the United States is 88 per 100,000 person-years. 15% of supraventricular arrhythmias are AFL and usually coexists with AF. More than 80% of patients who undergo RFA of typical AFL will have AF within the following 5 years. The incidence of AFL in men is more than twice that of women. Paroxysmal AFL can be seen in patients with no structural heart disease (SHD), whereas chronic AFL is frequently associated with underlying SHD, such as valvular disease or heart failure. Acute AFL may happen secondary to acute disease process, such as pericarditis, pulmonary embolism, exacerbation of lung disease, following heart or lung surgery, or myocardial infarction. [1]

3. Definition and classification

AFL is defined as abnormal atrial activity inside a reentrant circuit with a diameter more than 2 cm^2 at a high rate of 240–320 bpm which makes a continuous oscillation without an isoelectric baseline [2]. In contrast, focal atrial tachycardia (AT) is a rapid abnormal atrial rhythm originating from a "point source" with a baseline between P waves on ECG. The most practical classification is based on isthmus versus non-isthmus dependency (**Diagram 1**). According to the new classification, typical AFL is a macroreentrant atrial tachycardia that usually proceeds up the atrial septum (counterclockwise or CCW), down the lateral atrial wall, and through the CTI between the tricuspid valve annulus and inferior vena cava (IVC). It is also known as "common AFL" or "CTI-dependent AFL." When the circuit rotates in the opposite direction, it is referred to as clockwise (CW) typical AFL or reverse typical AFL (**Figure 1**). Clockwise AFL is observed in only 10% of clinical cases. However, the flutter wave morphology might change in the presence of underlying atrial disease, prior surgery, or previous ablation which makes the flutter wave morphology not a reliable indicator of AFL type [2, 3].

Atypical flutter, or "non-CTI-dependent macroreentrant atrial tachycardia," is attributed to those flutters that do not use the CTI originating in the right (RA) or left atrium (LA) [3]. In this

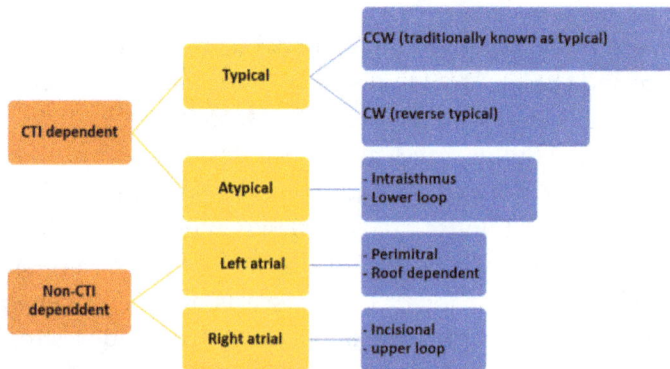

Diagram 1. Classification of atrial flutter (see the text for discussion).

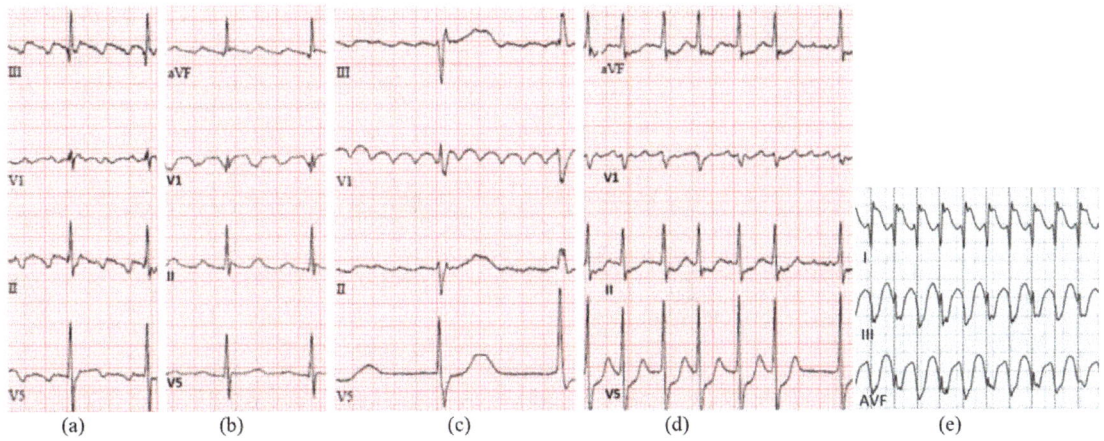

Figure 1. Counterclockwise typical flutter (a), clockwise typical flutter (b), atypical flutter (c), atrial fibrillation (d), atrial flutter 1:1 in a patient on flecainide (e). In tracing d, the atrial waves amplitude in V1 is changing with irregular irregular RR interval.

group, different circuits have been described, including "perimitral flutter" reentry, LA roof dependent flutter and reentry around scars from previous surgery or ablation in atria. Obviously, these flutters are not amenable to ablation of the CTI, but common AFL often coexists with these atypical reentry circuits [4].

3.1. Anatomy of the CTI

The CTI is bounded anteriorly by the tricuspid annulus and posteriorly by the ostium of the IVC and the eustachian ridge. The width and muscle thickness of CTI are variable, from several millimeters to around 3 cm in width and depth of 1 cm roughly. The CTI is wider in the lateral portion and thinner in the central portion. The central isthmus is concave and pouch-like in 47 and 45% of patients, respectively. The subeustachian isthmus is the area between the tricuspid annulus and the eustachian ridge which ends in IVC junction. The pectinates, spare the myocardium just in atrial part of the tricuspid valve and makes the smooth portion of the CTI which is referred to as the vestibular portion. Of note, the septal part of the CTI is adjacent to the posterior extensions of the AV node as well as the middle cardiac vein [5, 6]. This anatomic proximity explains the higher risk of AV block if ablation is done in the septal aspect. Also, the smooth vestibular portion around the tricuspid valve lies very close to the right coronary artery.

4. Clinical manifestation

The patients with flutter sometimes are asymptomatic or may present with a variety of symptoms including palpitations, dyspnea, fatigue, dizziness or reduced functional class. However, it might be the first presentation of more serious conditions like acute pulmonary embolism, acute coronary syndrome or acute pulmonary edema. The severity of symptoms closely depends on the baseline left ventricular ejection fraction (LVEF), ventricular rate during the flutter and underlying SHD. As a common scenario, the patients present with a stroke or with decompensated heart failure secondary to tachycardia-induced cardiomyopathy. AFL occurs in nearly 25% of patients with AF.

5. Management

5.1. Acute management

The clinical presentation will dictate acute therapeutic approach which may include cardioversion or rate control strategy. Cardioversion (electrical or chemical) is usually the initial treatment of choice. Antiarrhythmic medication such as intravenous amiodarone, sotalol, have been reported with a high success rate of chemical cardioversion. These class III antiarrhythmics prolong the refractory period leading slower cycle length which could terminate AFL. Interestingly, intravenous ibutilide has been more effective than the formers up to 76% of patients. Electrical cardioversion at a low energy of 50 J has very high success rate. Overdrive atrial pacing by a catheter in RA or in preexisting pacemaker/defibrillator is an effective alternative option in terminating typical AFL. Anticoagulation by using the same criteria as for AF, prior to cardioversion should be considered [3]. In order to control the rate, oral or intravenous atrioventricular node (AVN) blockers such as verapamil, diltiazem, beta blockers, and digoxin, can be used. However, the rate control is difficult to achieve as opposed to AF.

5.2. Chronic management

If AFL occurs in the context of an acute disease process, long-term rhythm control medication is usually not required once the AFL is converted and the underlying pathologic process is eliminated. However, if there is a certain substrate for AFL recurrence such as enlarged RA or scar, medical suppression of AFL can be extremely difficult. Hence, the ablation procedure with highly successful rate and low complication risk is the approach of choice for typical AFL [7]. However, medication may be tried in some situation (i.e. patient preference). Several antiarrhythmic drugs have been somehow effective in AFL suppression, including class IC (flecainide and propafenone), and class III (usually sotalol and amiodarone) antiarrhythmics. In the absence of SHD, class IC agents are the first line medication. The antiarrhythmic agents should be combined with AVN blockers to avoid the risk of rapid ventricular rates. In fact, class IC drugs have a vagolytic effect on AVN. Although the atrial flutter rate will be slowed, more proportion of these atrial impulses will be conducted through AVN (enhanced conduction), by which net ventricular rate increases [3]. As a result, rapid 1:1 AV conduction is mostly seen if Class IC antiarrhythmic medication is not combined with AVN blockers such as beta blockers (**Figure 1e**). As mentioned, typical AFL is very amenable to ablation but AV junction ablation and pacemaker implantation may be indicated if rhythm and rate control strategies including ablation have failed in atypical flutter. The anticoagulant policy will be implemented based on the same guideline for AF.

6. Typical flutter

6.1. Electrocardiographic characteristics

In "typical" counterclockwise AFL, the wave of depolarization propagates through the lateral right atrium, then travels through the CTI in a lateral-to-medial direction. The wave of depolarization arrives at the inferior part of the interatrial septum, splits and propagates caudocephalically up the septum, finally traveling across the roof to arrive lateral RA to complete the circuit. At the same time, the depolarization wave propagates from inferior septum to the lateral wall of the left atrium. Flutter waves have constant morphology and polarity with same CL. In typical AFL, they are most visible in lead V1 and the inferior leads (II, III, aVF) with a sawtooth appearance. The propagation of depolarization wave is through interatrial septum which makes it positive or negative in inferior leads in clockwise (high to low) or counterclockwise (low to high) AFL, respectively. The wave includes a slow downsloping portion, with a sharp negative deflection, followed by a rapid positive deflection, merging to the next downsloping deflection (**Figure 2**). Because of constant activation inside the circuit, there is no electrically silent period and consequently no isoelectric period. This is as opposed to focal AT with silent periods between focal discharges (**Figure 3**). However, focal

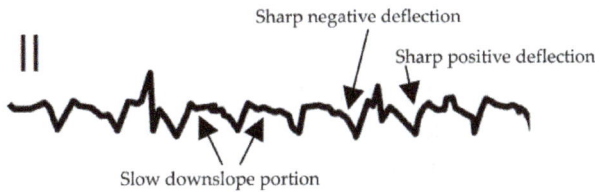

Figure 2. The typical CCW flutter ECG characteristic (see the text).

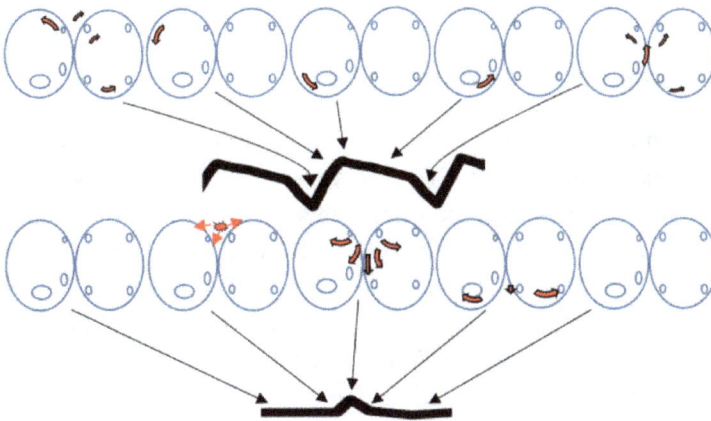

Figure 3. The top diagram demonstrates the atrial activation sequence correlated with typical CCW atrial flutter. The slow conduction through CTI causes the flatter portion of flutter wave. The bottom diagram shows atrial activation sequence in focal AT with silent periods causing flat isoelectric line.

AT can produce a continuous wave pattern on ECG if the atrial CL is short enough to shorten the interval between atrial depolarization [4, 8].

During CW AFL, the positive deflections in the inferior leads are nearly equal negative deflections in inferior leads making a sinusoidal pattern which makes it somehow difficult to recognize positive from negative deflections. So lead V1 is important in order to recognize clockwise typical AFL.

The atrial rate in AFL is typically 240–320 bpm, but it might be slower if conduction is slow inside the circuit due to scars from prior ablation or surgery. Also, antiarrhythmic medication can cause conduction delay. In these instances, distinct isoelectric intervals between flutter waves may be recognized similar to focal AT. The rapid ventricular response is occasionally seen in those patients with underlying anterogradely conducting bypass tracts or secondary to high sympathetic tone (e.g., exercise, sympathomimetic drugs) which enhance AV conduction [2]. Typically, the patients with flutter present with 2:1 AV conduction but variable AV conduction and higher grade AV block (e.g., 4:1 or 6:1) or AV dissociation (slow and fixed RR interval) may occur. P wave morphology is usually of limited anatomical value for precise circuit localization in other atypical forms of AFL. If there is any doubt on the initial ECG, infusion of adenosine or carotid massage may transiently decrease AV conduction, unmasking the flutter waves. Adenosine and digoxin increase the degree of AV block, but shorten atrial refractoriness and can cause the AFL to degenerate into AF. Of note, AF is sometimes confused with AFL when the atrial activity in lead V1 might look organized (see **Figure 1d**).

In case of AF, the cycle length of atrial waves is less than 200 ms, the RR interval is truly irregular (with precise measurement) and atrial activation is not usually organized in the limb leads. Also, there is no true relationship between the apparent "flutter waves" and QRS complexes, best seen in lead V1, and close inspection often reveals the atrial waves do not have the constant morphology and amplitude as seen in a real atrial flutter. These instances are usually defined as "coarse AF." In rare examples, RA is in AFL but LA is in AF in which lead V1 might show more uniform morphology but the other leads manifest characteristics of fibrillation [9].

6.2. Electrophysiological testing in typical flutter

In brief, RFA is performed by creating lesions across the critical isthmus to achieve the complete and stable bi-directional block across CTI. The procedure includes linear lesion, finding the residual conducting gaps to eliminate, and ultimately the end point is the confirmation of bidirectional block across CTI. Typically, three catheters are used for ablation of typical AFL. They include the ablation catheter, multipolar coronary sinus (CS) catheter, and a duo-decapolar halo catheter. Halo catheter is positioned around tricuspid annulus so that proximal poles positioned in upper interatrial septum and roof, mid poles positioned from high to low in the lateral RA anterior to the crista terminalis and distal poles positioned in lateral inferior at 6–7 o'clock in the LAO view in fluoroscopy. In fact, the distal poles will record the middle and lateral part of the CTI [10, 11].

6.2.1. Induction of tachycardia

It's very crucial to distinguish between isthmus-dependent and non-isthmus-dependent flutters in order to perform curative ablation. Hence, AFL should be induced to confirm the diagnosis and make sure the AFL is isthmus dependent prior to ablation. AFL can usually be induced with programmed electrical stimulation (PES) from different locations; however, it is usually performed with pacing from proximal coronary sinus which can induce CCW typical flutter. Isoproterenol infusion (0.5–4 µg/min) may be needed to facilitate tachycardia induction. Burst pacing or atrial extra stimulus at the shorter CL/ coupling intervals will more likely induce AF which is often self-terminating. However, AF can be sustained around 10% of cases needing cardioversion in EP lab. The importance of AF induction in these patients with no clinical history of AF is uncertain [10, 12].

6.2.2. Flutter circuit features

In typical AFL, intracardiac electrogram (EGM) shows bipolar electrograms with constant CL, polarity and morphology with sequential atrial activation characteristic of a macroreentry in which the atrial CL is very stable and less than <15% as opposed to focal AT [13]. The endocardial recordings of the interatrial septum, upper anterolateral, and CTI indicates low-voltage atrial electrical activity cover 100% of the tachycardia cycle length (TCL) (**Figure 4**). In focal AT, the atrial activation covers less than 50% of TCL, even if only RA atrial activation recordings are taken account. The CTI is the zone of delayed conduction required for establishing reentry. Some studies show slow conduction area is probably located in the medial part of CTI in older patients versus the lateral part of CTI in younger people [7, 14]. With consideration of depolarization propagation around the circuit in typical isthmus-dependent AFL, the atrial activation sequence is predictable. The onset of flutter waves in the surface ECG is simultaneous with activation of the septal atrial electrogram which is His atrial recording in clockwise and the atrial recording of proximal CS in counterclockwise AFL [9].

6.2.3. Diagnostic maneuvers

6.2.3.1. Entrainment and technique

Entrainment is the essential maneuver to confirm the diagnosis. It determines whether AFL is CTI dependent [12].

Overdrive atrial pacing is performed at a CL of 10–20 ms shorter than the TCL to entrain. As shown in **Figure 5**, if the pacing site is farther from the reentrant circuit, it takes longer for the impulse to get the circuit and entrain the tachycardia. By definition, the entrainment is a continuous resetting of a reentrant circuit with an excitable gap by a series of stimuli with following characteristics:

1. During pacing at shorter CL, all P waves (and intracardiac atrial electrograms) are accelerated to the pacing rate

2. During pacing at progressively faster cycle lengths, progressive fusion of flutter waves (surface ECG) or intracardiac EGM occurs

3. The same tachycardia (same TCL and atrial activation sequence) resumes upon termination of pacing.

The post-pacing interval (PPI) is the time between the last pacing stimulus that entrained the AFL and the next recorded atrial EGM at the same pacing site (same catheter through which

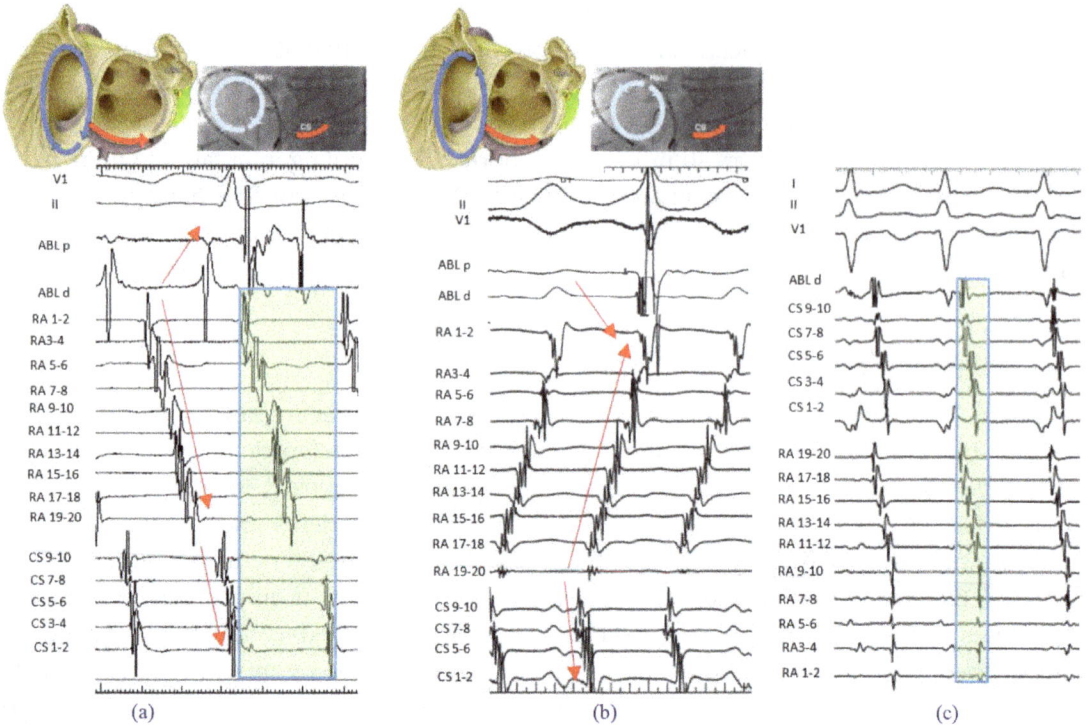

Figure 4. Electrocardiogram and endocardial electrogram of CCW typical flutter (b), CW (reverse) typical flutter (a) and focal atrial tachycardia (c). Arrows show the atrial activation sequence. The halo catheter (RA channel)) has 10 bipolar electrograms recorded from the distal (low lateral right atrium or RA 1–2) to the proximal (high right atrium or RA 19–20) poles of the halo catheter positioned around the tricuspid annulus. The distal pole of RA 1–2 is at 7 o'clock and the proximal pole of RA 19–20 is at 1–2 o'clock. CS 9–10 electrograms are recorded from the CS proximal positioned at the CS ostium, ABL d (distal) electrogram is recorded from ablation catheter positioned in the cavotricuspid isthmus. Green shading shows the portion of the tachycardia cycle covered by the activation; which is around 100% in atrial flutter and less than 50% in focal atrial tachycardia (see the text).

pacing was done). Obviously, PPI will be shorter if the pacing stimulus site is closer to the circuit. Accordingly, if PPI is equal or within 20 ms of TCL, it means the pacing stimulus site is inside the circuit. In order to assess whether AFL is isthmus (CTI) dependent, an ablation catheter is placed in CTI and paced at shorter CL to entrain AFL. If PPI is within 20 ms of TCL, it indicates that CTI is in the circuit which confirms AFL is isthmus (CTI) dependent. If the pacing site is outside of the circuit, the PPI will be equal to TCL plus the time required for the stimulus to travel from the pacing site to the flutter circuit and return back to the stimulus site [12, 14, 15] (**Figure 5**).

6.3. Ablation

6.3.1. Technique

Typically, a 4-mm irrigated steerable ablation catheter is used in order to deliver point-by-point RF applications across CTI. Adequacy and quality of lesions depend on proper contact, local

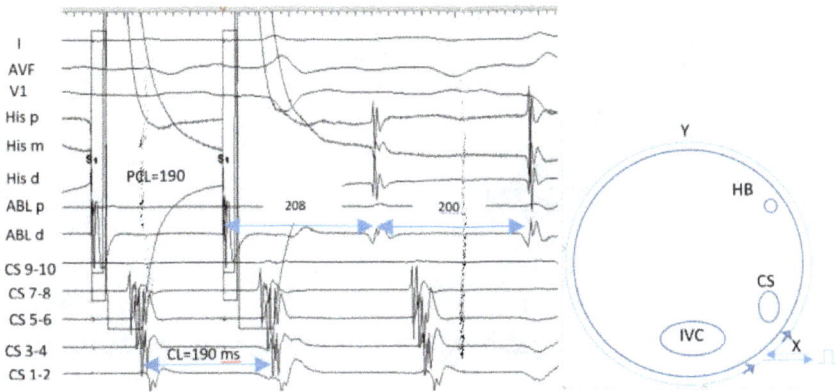

Figure 5. The right diagram illustrates the entrainment concept. The time from the stimulus site to the circuit is equal to X. The whole circuit time is equal to Y, so the time required for the stimulus to travel from stimulus site to get the circuit, turn around the circuit, returning back to the stimulus site is equal to 2X + Y. In the left tracing, TCL =200, overdrive pacing from ablation catheter positioned at CTI is performed at CL = 190 ms which entrains the tachycardia. The PPI (208 ms in this example) is measured from the stimulus to the first potential appears in ablation catheter channel. PPI-TCL = 8 ms which confirms the ablation catheter is inside the circuit at the CTI; hence, the flutter is CTI dependent.

blood flow, enough power, and tissue thickness. A guiding sheath (e.g. SR0 or ramp sheath) can help stabilizing the catheter position and prevent sliding off the line of ablation during RF application. At first, the catheter is advanced into the RV in RAO view, then is dragged back gradually until the EGM shows small atrial and large ventricular electrograms. The relative electrogram size of the ventricular and atrial signals helps to estimate the approximate location of catheter tip (e.g. the A/V ratio is around 1:4 at the ventricular side of the tricuspid annulus, and 4:1 near the IVC). The tip of the ablation catheter is finely adjusted in midway between the interatrial septum (CS Ostium as a landmark) and lateral RA lateral in the LAO view (at around 6 or 7 o'clock). The first RF application is delivered at the tricuspid annulus with small AV ratio. After each RF application lasting for 30–60 s, the atrial electrogram voltage is reduced and may become fragmented; then the catheter is dragged back around 4 mm until EGM shows new sharp atrial electrogram (not far field), and the next RF burn is delivered. This sequence is repeated until EGM shows minimal or no atrial electrograms which implies that the catheter tip has reached the IVC border [10, 16, 17].

6.3.2. Anatomic considerations

Firstly, the eustachian ridge is a "floppy" structure that comprises the posterior border of CTI and separates the IVC from the inferior RA, and sometimes prevents complete ablation of the posterior part of CTI with simple dragging of the catheter. In such situation, the catheter tip should be curled back, in order to get access to the most posterior part of CTI and the floor of pouch created by "Eustachian ridge"(**Figure 6**). It is important to keep in mind that AV block can occur in approximately 1% of cases, particularly during ablation of the medial side of CTI (5 o'clock) which is close to the septum. Observation of changing variable conduction of 2:1–3:1 or appearance of relatively regular QRS complexes should warrant possibility of damage to

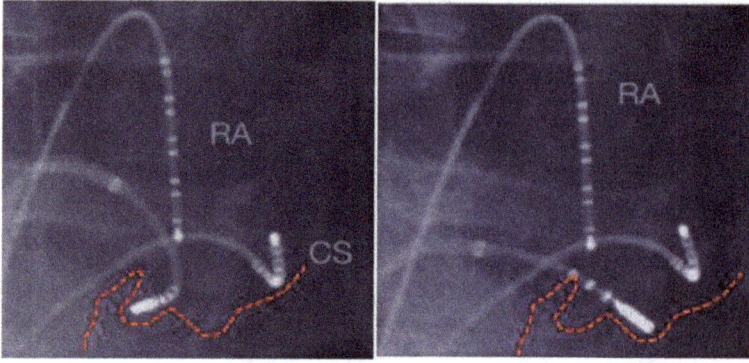

Figure 6. In some difficult cases, the eustachian ridge separates the IVC from the inferior RA and creates a pouch. In order to get access to the pouch floor to complete the line of the block, the ablation catheter should be curled back as shown on the left panel.

AVN and consequent high-grade AV block. So the risk of AV block is less likely if ablation is done far away septum [18, 19]. In AFL recurrence and re-do cases, 3D mapping system and intracardiac echocardiography will be helpful to figure out the complex anatomy and hence to ablate effectively the gaps.

6.4. Post-ablation study

6.4.1. Identification and ablation of residual gaps

With respect to isthmus anatomy and the presence of potential pouches, conduction gaps frequently remain despite continuous lesions. Locating and ablating residual gaps is mandatory to achieve complete bidirectional block and to prevent AFL recurrence. The residual gaps can be detected via local electrograms including fractionated EGM potential or the isoelectric interval between double potentials [20] (**Figure 7**).

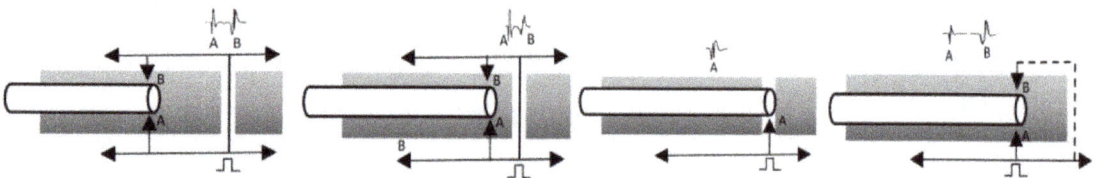

Figure 7. Identification of residual gaps in the ablation line. An interval separating the two components of double potentials recorded along the ablation line in the CTI during CS pacing, after RF ablation. The first component (potential a) is produced once the stimulus impulse reaches the one side of the ablation catheter. If there is a gap along the line of ablation, the impulse still can travel through the gap to another side of the ablation catheter, producing second potential (B). When the tip of catheter moves toward to the site of the gap, the time required for an impulse to reach the tip of the catheter on the other side gets shorter, which leads to shortening of the interval between two components. Finally, at the site of gap, the two signals will be fused and the double potentials disappear. This approach with moving the catheter through the line can detect the gap. The last diagram shows completion of block line in which the impulse should turn around the RA (far away CTI) that will obviously increase the time required for the impulse to reach spot B; thus, the interval between two components will be prolonged.

6.4.2. Endpoints

Confirmation of bidirectional block is traditionally considered as the endpoint of AFL ablation. The created lesion can recover conduction so bidirectional block should be verified with the current maneuver as the endpoint of RF ablation and repeated after 20–30 min monitoring [21].

6.4.3. Atrial activation sequence during atrial pacing in the presence of isthmus block

Pacing from the medial side of the ablation line (e.g. from CS proximal) is performed and atrial activation sequence is evaluated (**Figure 8**). In the presence of medial to lateral block across

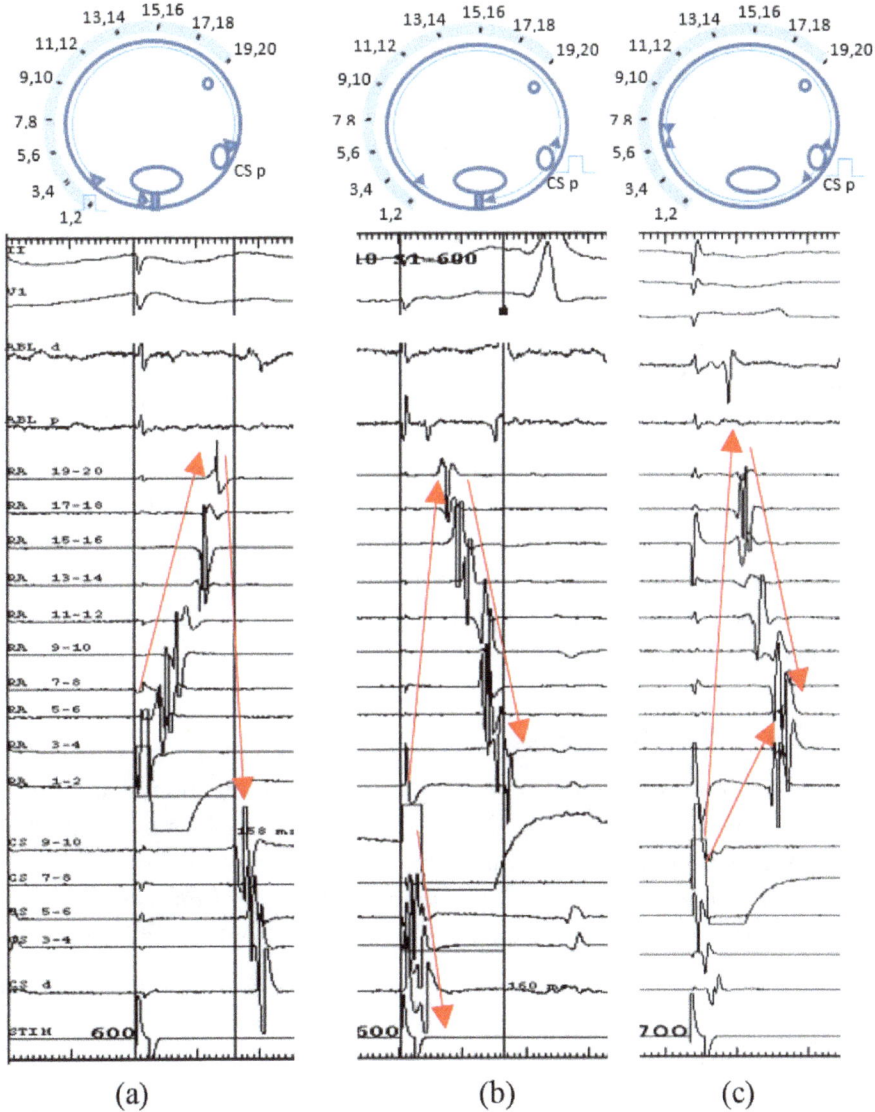

Figure 8. Right atrial endocardial electrograms recorded during CSp pacing from distal halo catheter or RA 1–2 after ablation (a) and from CSp pacing before (c) and after (b) ablation of CTI during sinus rhythm (see the text for discussion).

CTI, atrial depolarization wave must propagate caudocephalically up the septum and travel down to the lateral RA to arrive at distal poles of halo catheter. So the distal poles of halo catheter are the last poles which record the atrial potentials (**Figure 8b**). In order to assess the lateral to medial block across CTI, pacing from lateral to the ablation line is performed (e.g. halo distal poles or tip of ablation catheter at 8:00 o'clock). In case of lateral to medial block, atrial depolarization wave will propagate superiorly up the lateral RA and travel down the interatrial septum to reach the CS ostium, recorded at proximal CS (**Figure 8a**). **Figure 8c** shows the atrial activation during CS proximal pacing prior to medial to lateral isthmus block which demonstrates the collision of the cranial and caudal right atrial wave fronts in the mid-lateral RA (RA 5–6).

6.4.4. Trans CTI conduction time

CS proximal or low lateral RA is usually paced in order to measure conduction interval across CTI. Obviously, the interval is the time from the stimulus pacing artifact from one side of the isthmus (e.g. CS proximal) to the atrial electrogram recorded on the other side (e.g. distal halo poles). More than 50% prolongation of this interval or an absolute interval time of 150 ms or more is in favor of CTI block [22, 23].

6.4.5. Differential pacing

This maneuver is used to assess CW and CCW block across CTI. At first, pacing is performed close to the ablation line, then pacing site is moved away from first pacing spot (**Figure 9**). For example, to check CCW (lateral to medial) block, the pacing is done from halo distal poles (Halo 1,2) and the time from stimulus artifact to the atrial electrogram recorded on the proximal CS is measured. Then pacing site is done farther from ablation line (Halo 3,4). If there is CCW, the measured interval will be shortened on the latter spot (Halo 3,4). When CTI conduction is intact, conduction occurs via a counterclockwise wavefront across the CTI to reach proximal CS, so the measured interval will be longer once it is paced from Halo 3,4 compared to Halo 1,2 [24].

6.4.6. Electroanatomical mapping

Electroanatomical 3D mapping can also be used to confirm conduction block across CTI. For example, when CCW block is present, Halo 1,2 pacing results in an activation wavefront directing in a CW pattern and CTI immediately medial to the ablation line will be the last part in the circuit which will be activated. If CTI is intact, with pacing from Halo 1,2 the activation wavefront travels rapidly through the CTI, with the upper septum will be the last part of activation.

6.5. Complication

RF ablation of the typical AFL is relatively safe, with an average complication rate of 3% which includes mostly peripheral vascular injury (0.5%). The risk of serious complication is very low which include complete heart block (0.3%), tamponade, myocardial infarction due to damage to the right coronary artery, stroke and pulmonary embolism (0.1%). The recurrence

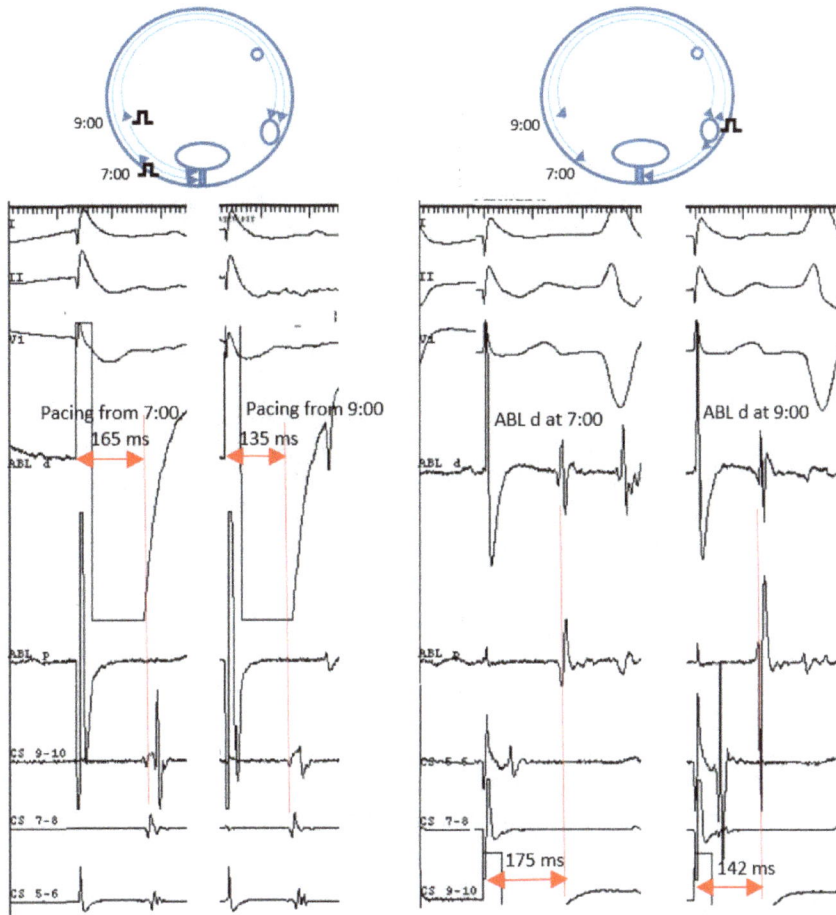

Figure 9. The method of differential pacing to evaluate bidirectional CTI block (see the text).

rate of AFL has been reduced by using irrigated tip catheters and is around half of the recurrence in standard RF ablation (7 vs 14%). The occurrence of AF or atypical AFL is dramatically high at around 70% in long-term follow up [25, 26]

7. Atypical AFL

Atypical AFL frequently demonstrates attenuated flutter waves which help to distinguish from typical flutter. They are classified as atypical right or left atrial flutter [27] (**Figure 10**). Prompt identification of these AFL types will maximize the success rate of ablation.

7.1. Atypical right atrial isthmus-dependent flutter

7.1.1. Lower loop reentry

Lower loop reentry is a form of CTI-dependent AFL in which the circuit is around IVC. The eustachian ridge and lower crista terminalis usually cause a breakdown in wavefront

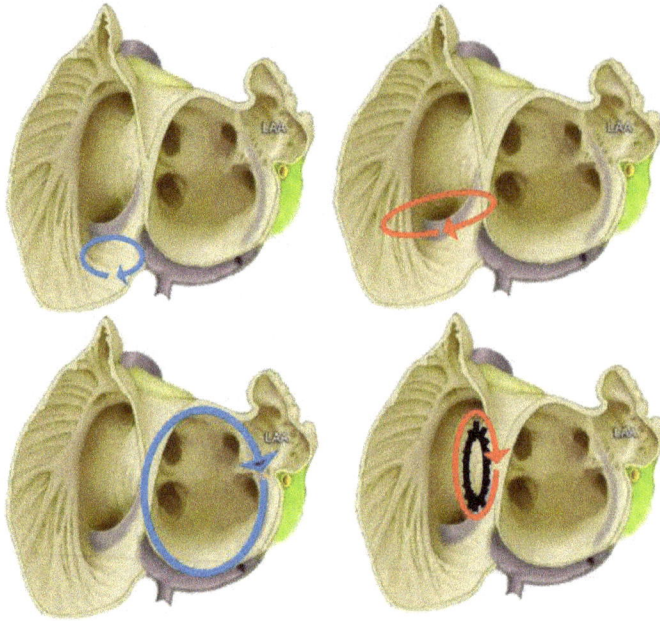

Figure 10. Types of atypical flutter. Top left, Intraisthmus reentry. Top right, lower loop reentry. Bottom left, perimitral reentry. Bottom right, incisional (around ASD patch) reentry.

conduction across CTI; consequently, impulse revolves around the IVC instead of the tricuspid annulus. It is mostly identified during 3D activation mapping [28].

7.1.2. Intraisthmus reentry

The circuit of intraisthmus reentry is bounded by the medial side of CTI and CS ostium. The previous ablation at the CTI might predispose and perpetuate this reentry. The EGMs are usually similar to typical AFL but entrainment shows the lateral CTI is not inside the circuit (long PPI) whereas the medial side of CTI presents in the circuit (short PPI). The mapping of the region between proximal CS and medial CTI usually shows fractionated or double potentials which are a good target for ablation. A linear lesion across the medial CTI usually breaks the circuit [27, 28].

7.2. Atypical right atrial non-isthmus dependent flutter

7.2.1. Lesional right atrial flutter

These circuits arise around a low-voltage area, incision, patch or scar in the lateral or posterolateral RA. These areas usually develop after the atriotomy and surgery for the congenital disease. 3D activation mapping is an excellent modality to identify this type of AFL circuits [28].

7.2.2. Upper loop reentry

In this type of AFL, the wavefront activation propagates around the superior vena cava (SVC) and travels through a conduction gap in the crista terminalis.

7.2.3. Dual-loop reentry

The coexistence of two circuits is known as dual-loop reentry. The activation wavefront can propagate through both circuits intermittently. In practice, they are identified when the ablation of one circuit leads to change in atrial activation sequence suggesting a transition to the other circuit [27].

7.3. Atypical left atrial flutter

LA flutter often coexists with AF. It is usually secondary to AF ablation (up to 50%) or open heart surgery for the valvular disease. The central obstacle of the AFL circuits is low-voltage or scar areas in the LA detected by electroanatomic 3D mapping [29].

7.3.1. ECG characteristics of left atrial flutter

Whenever the flutter wave morphology in ECG is not characteristic of typical AFL, left atrial flutter must be considered. A characteristic finding in LA flutter is a dominantly positive broad deflection in lead V1. The combination of attenuated deflections in the frontal leads with a dominantly positive deflection in V1 also suggests that origin of flutter is probably in LA. Uncommonly, negative flutter deflections in the inferior leads might be seen in left AFL mimicking typical AFL (pseudo-typical flutter). However, typical AFL demonstrates positive overshoot immediately following the negative deflection. This positive deflection is as a result of inferiorly down activation of the lateral RA. Lack of this sharp positive deflection raises suspicion of atypical AFL. In the presence of low voltage areas, the electrical impulse traversing the isthmus (protected within scar) might generate low voltage potentials, demonstrated on the surface ECG as an iso-electric interval. In addition, a small portion of the atria is being activated during the silent isoelectric period. Therefore, the isoelectric interval strongly supports the presence of a slow conducting isthmus, although its absence does not exclude it. For example, if intracardiac CS electrograms coincide with an isoelectric interval, it suggests CS region may be involved in the reentrant circuit, indirectly implies the flutter might be left sided in origin. Likewise, the electrograms of CTI region coincide with the isoelectric period between the negative flutter waves in typical AFL [30, 31].

7.3.2. Perimitral atrial flutter

In this type of AFL, the reentrant circuit arises around the mitral annulus. 3D voltage mapping often shows low-voltage or scar areas on the posterior LA which act as a boundary of this circuit. Most of the patients have a past history of AF ablation [29].

7.4. EPS and mapping in atypical AFL

In addition to CS and Halo catheter, the transseptal puncture is performed to insert a catheter in LA (usually irrigated tip ablation catheter) for the full study. In order to confirm LA flutter, a systematic approach is used. The first step is the exclusion of CTI dependent AFL. Coronary sinus activation from proximal to distal can suggest that AFL origin is from the RA; however, CS activation sequences are not very valuable in LA flutter diagnosis. If EGMs recorded throughout RA (i.e. atrial electrograms recorded on all Halo poles) covers more than 50% of the TCL, it is another clue for RA AFL. Another helpful maneuver is entrainment at multiple sites in the RA and comparison of their PPIs. For instance, if PPI is shorter in septum compared to lateral RA or CTI, it might be suggestive for LA flutter. In fact, the gradient of PPI in LA flutter typically is longest (more than 30 ms) in the lateral RA and remarkably shorter in the mid and distal coronary sinus. However, roof or anterior LA flutter might show long PPI in mid to distal CS [28, 29, 32]. The 3D mapping system is often necessary to perform the full activation and voltage mapping for localization and effective ablation of the reentrant circuit [33].

8. Conclusion

Atrial flutter is relatively common atrial arrhythmia with the nearly similar morbidity and mortality to atrial fibrillation. However, it's highly amenable to RF ablation. This procedure has emerged as therapy of choice in the light of highly successful rate and low complication risk. The knowledge of the anatomy and electrophysiology of the atrial flutter circuit is essential to choosing the optimal site for elimination of reentry. An electroanatomic 3D mapping system is highly recommended to perform the full activation and voltage mapping in order to localize the circuit and critical isthmus targeted for effective ablation.

Acknowledgements

I thank my wife, Mojgan for her continued inspiration and my daughter, Diana for her tremendous support to complete this chapter. But most importantly, I want to thank my son Arshia for his great technical support and his help, editing this chapter.

Disclosure

None.

Author details

Hamid Reza Bonakdar

Address all correspondence to: hamidreza.bonakdar@gmail.com

St. Michael Hospital, Affiliated to University of Toronto, Canada

References

[1] Granada J, Uribe W, Chyou PH, Maassen K, Vierkant R, Smith PN, et al. Incidence and predictors of atrial flutter in the general population. Journal of the American College of Cardiology. 2000 Dec;**36**(7):2242-2246. DOI: 10.1016/S0735-1097(00)00982-7

[2] Saoudi N, Cosi'o F, Waldo A, Chen SA, Iesaka Y, Lesh M, et al. A classification of atrial flutter and regular atrial tachycardia according to electrophysiologic mechanism and anatomic bases. A statement from a joint expert group from the working Group of Arrhythmias of the European Society of Cardiology and the north American society of pacing and electrophysiology. European Heart Journal. 2001;**22**:1162-1182. DOI: 10.1053/euhj.2001.2658

[3] Blomstrom-Lundqvist C, Scheinman MM, Aliot EM, et al. ACC/AHA/ESC guidelines for the management of patients with supraventricular arrhythmias–executive summary. A report of the American college of cardiology/American heart association task force on practice guidelines and the European society of cardiology committee for practice guidelines (writing committee to develop guidelines for the management of patients with supraventricular arrhythmias) developed in collaboration with NASPE-Heart Rhythm Society. Journal of the American College of Cardiology. 2003;**42**:1493-1531. DOI: 10.1161/01.CIR.0000091380.04100.84

[4] January CT, Wann LS, Alpert JS, et al. 2014 AHA/ACC/HRS guideline for the management of patients with atrial fibrillation: A report of the American College of Cardiology/American Heart Association task force on practice guidelines and the Heart Rhythm Society. Journal of the American College of Cardiology. 2014 Dec 2;**64**(21):e1-76. DOI: 10.1016/j.jacc.2014.03.021

[5] Tai CT, Chen SA. Cavotricuspid isthmus: Anatomy, electrophysiology, and long-term outcome of radiofrequency ablation. Pacing and Clinical Electrophysiology. 2009;**32**: 1591-1595. DOI: 10.1111/j.1540-8159.2009.02555.x

[6] Saremi F, Pourzand L, Krishnan S, et al. Right atrial cavotricuspid isthmus: Anatomic characterization with multi-detector row CT. Radiology. 2008;**247**:658-668. DOI: 10.1148/radiol.2473070819

[7] Waldo AL, Atiezna F. Atrial flutter: Mechanisms, features, and management. In: Zipes DP, Jalife J, editors. Cardiac Electrophysiology: From Cell to Bedside. 5th ed. Philadelphia: Saunders; 2009. pp. 567-576

[8] Medi C, Kalman JM. Prediction of the atrial flutter circuit location from the surface electrocardiogram. Europace. 2008;**10**:786-796. DOI: 10.1093/europace/eun106

[9] Josephson ME. Atrial flutter. In: Zimetbaum P, Josephson M, editors. Practical Clinical Electrophysiology. 2nd ed. Wolter Kluwer; 2017. pp. 73-83

[10] Josephson ME. Atrial flutter and fibrillation. In: Josephson ME, editor. Clinical Cardiac Electrophysiology. 4th ed. Philadelphia: Lippincott Williams & Wilkins; 2008. pp. 285-338

[11] Miyazaki H, Stevenson WG, Stephenson K, et al. Entrainment mapping for rapid distinction of left and right atrial tachycardias. Heart Rhythm. 2006;3:516-523. DOI: 10.1016/j. hrthm.2006.01.014

[12] Deo R, Berger R. The clinical utility of entrainment pacing. Journal of Cardiovascular Electrophysiology. 2009;20:466-470. DOI: 10.1111/j.1540-8167.2008.01409.x

[13] Jaïs P, Matsuo S, Knecht S, Weerasooriya R, Hocini M, et al. A deductive mapping strategy for atrial tachycardia following atrial fibrillation ablation: Importance of localized reentry. Journal of Cardiovascular Electrophysiology. 2009;(5):480-491. DOI: 10.1111/ j.1540-8167.2008.01373.x

[14] Huang JL, Tai CT, Lin YJ, et al. Right atrial substrate properties associated with age in patients with typical atrial flutter. Heart Rhythm. 2008;5:1144-1151. DOI: 10.1016/j. hrthm.2008.05.009

[15] Waldo AL. Atrial flutter: Entrainment characteristics. Journal of Cardiovascular Electrophysiology. 1997 Mar;8(3):337-352. DOI: 10.1111/j.1540-8167.1997.tb00798.x

[16] Marrouche NF, Schweikert R, Saliba W, et al. Use of different catheter ablation technologies for treatment of typical atrial flutter: Acute results and long-term follow-up. Pacing and Clinical Electrophysiology. 2003;26:743-746. DOI: 10.1046/j.1460-9592.2003.00126.x

[17] Cosio FG, Pastor A, Nunez A, Giocolea A. Catheter ablation of typical atrial flutter. In: Zipes DP, Haissaguerre M, editors. Catheter Ablation of Arrhythmias. Armonk, NY: Futura; 2002. pp. 131-152

[18] Gami AS, Edwards WD, Lachman N, et al. Electrophysiological anatomy of typical atrial flutter: The posterior boundary and causes for difficulty with ablation. Journal of Cardiovascular Electrophysiology. 2010;21:144-149. DOI: 10.1111/j.1540-8167.2009.01607.x

[19] Lo LW, Tai CT, Lin YJ, et al. Characteristics of the cavotricuspid isthmus in predicting recurrent conduction in the long-term follow-up. Journal of Cardiovascular Electrophysiology. 2009;20:39-43. DOI: 10.1111/j.1540-8167.2008.01269.x

[20] Shah D, Haïssaguerre M, Jaïs P, Takahashi A, Hocini M, Clémenty J. High-density mapping of activation through an incomplete isthmus ablation line. Circulation. 1999;2: 211-215. PMID: 9892585

[21] Chen J, De Chillou C, Basiouny T, Sadoul N, Filho JD, Magnin-Poull I. et al, Cavotricuspid isthmus mapping to assess bidirectional block during common atrial flutter radiofrequency ablation. Circulation. 1999 Dec 21-28;100(25):2507-2513. DOI: 10.1161/01. CIR.100.25.2507

[22] Chen J, De Chillou C, Hoff PI, Rossvoll O, Andronache M, Sadoul N, et al. Identification of extremely slow conduction in the cavotricuspid isthmus during common atrial flutter

ablation. Journal of Interventional Cardiac Electrophysiology : An International Journal of Arrhythmias and Pacing. 2002 Aug;7(1):67-75. DOI: 10.1023/A:102082430

[23] Oral H, Sticherling C, Tada H, et al. Role of transisthmus intervals in predicting bidirectional block after ablation of typical atrial flutter. Journal of Cardiovascular Electrophysiology. 2001;12:169-174. DOI: 10.1046/j.1540-8167.2001.00169.x

[24] Shah D, Haïssaguerre M, Takahashi A, et al. Differential pacing for distinguishing block from persistent conduction through an ablation line. Circulation. 2000;102:1517-1522. DOI: 10.1161/01.CIR.102.13.1517

[25] Gilligan DM, Zakaib JS, Fuller I, et al. Long-term outcome of patients after successful radiofrequency ablation for typical atrial flutter. Pacing and Clinical Electrophysiology. 2003;26:53-58. DOI: 10.1046/j.1460-9592.2003.00150.x

[26] Tai CT, Chen SA, Chiang CE, et al. Long-term outcome of radiofrequency catheter ablation for typical atrial flutter: Risk prediction of recurrent arrhythmias. Journal of Cardiovascular Electrophysiology. 1998;9:115-121. DOI: 10.1111/j.1540-8167.1998.tb00892.x

[27] Garan H. Atypical atrial flutter. Heart Rhythm. 2008;5:618-621. DOI: 10.1016/j.hrthm.2007.10.031

[28] Fiala M, Chovancik J, Neuwirth R, et al. Atrial macroreentry tachycardia in patients without obvious structural heart disease or previous cardiac surgical or catheter intervention: Characterization of arrhythmogenic substrates, reentry circuits, and results of catheter ablation. Journal of Cardiovascular Electrophysiology. 2007;18:824-832. DOI: 10.1111/j.1540-8167.2007.00859.x

[29] Morady F, Oral H, Chugh A. Diagnosis and ablation of atypical atrial tachycardia and flutter complicating atrial fibrillation ablation. Heart Rhythm. 2009;6(Suppl):S29-S32. DOI: 10.1016/j.hrthm.2009.02.011

[30] Shah D. ECG manifestations of left atrial flutter. Current Opinion in Cardiology. 2009;(1):35-41. DOI: 10.1097/HCO.0b013e32831ca5a8

[31] Bochoeyer A, Yang Y, Cheng J, Randall J. Surface electrocardiographic characteristics of right and left atrial flutter. Circulation. 2003;108:60-66. DOI: 10.1161/01.CIR.0000079140.35025.1E

[32] Jaïs P, Shah DC, Haïssaguerre M, Hocini M, Peng JT, et al. Mapping and ablation of left atrial flutters. Circulation. 2000;(25):2928-2934. DOI: 10.1161/01.CIR.101.25.2928

[33] Shah DC, Jais P, Haissaguerre M, Chouairi S, Takahashi A, Hocini M, et al. Three dimensional mapping of the common atrial flutter circuit in the right atrium. Circulation. 1997;96:3904-3912. DOI: 10.1161/01.CIR.96.11.3904

Brugada Type 1 Pattern and Risk Stratification for Sudden Death: Does the Key Hide in the ECG Analysis?

Antoine Deliniere, Francis Bessiere, Adrien Moreau,
Alexandre Janin, Gilles Millat and Philippe Chevalier

Abstract

Primary prevention of ventricular fibrillation is at the heart of the management of Brugada syndrome. Several recent studies have shown that the analysis of simple electrocardiographic criteria could help to stratify the risk of sudden death. In the present work, 12 markers were studied: spontaneous and permanent type 1 pattern, first-degree atrioventricular block, sinus node dysfunction, wide QRS in V2, aVR sign, fragmented QRS, S-waves in DI, early repolarization pattern, atrial fibrillation, type 1 in peripheral leads pattern, and long Tpeak-Tend interval. These electrical markers reflect abnormalities in conduction, depolarization, and repolarization that may indicate the severity of the disease. In this chapter, we carry out a review of these markers, their method of determination on the surface ECG, and the main studies highlighting their prognostic impact. We also review the main underlying pathophysiological hypotheses of Brugada syndrome.

Keywords: Brugada syndrome, Brugada type 1, primary prevention, risk stratification, ECG markers, ventricular fibrillation, sudden death

1. Introduction

Brugada syndrome is presumed to be a channelopathy causing sudden death by ventricular fibrillation. The diagnosis is based exclusively on the analysis of the surface electrocardiogram.

Today, the challenge is to improve the primary prevention of sudden death. There is a very large heterogeneity of ventricular fibrillation risk among patients and there is no reliable marker to assess this risk.

Beyond the diagnosis based on an accurate analysis of right precordial leads, the ECG phenotype of patients with Brugada syndrome is not unique. Many recent studies have shown that several electrocardiographic markers may indicate a more severe disease with an increased risk of sudden death.

A simple electrocardiographic approach to the risk of sudden death in Brugada syndrome may be worthwhile at a time when risk stratification is being questioned.

In this chapter, we propose to review the main ECG markers and the pathophysiological hypotheses underlying them.

2. Positive and differential diagnoses

2.1. Definition of Brugada type 1 pattern

The diagnosis of Brugada type 1 pattern is based exclusively on the analysis of the electrocardiogram. The panel of experts who elaborated the 2015 ESC recommendations on sudden death prevention [1] has reached a consensus on the diagnosis criteria.

Type 1 pattern is defined by a coved ST segment elevation with a rise of the J-point ≥2 mm in at least one derivation between V1 and V2 on a resting surface electrocardiogram (**Figure 1**). It is often accepted [2] that the T waves must be negative in the same lead(s), although this criterion is not included in the guidelines.

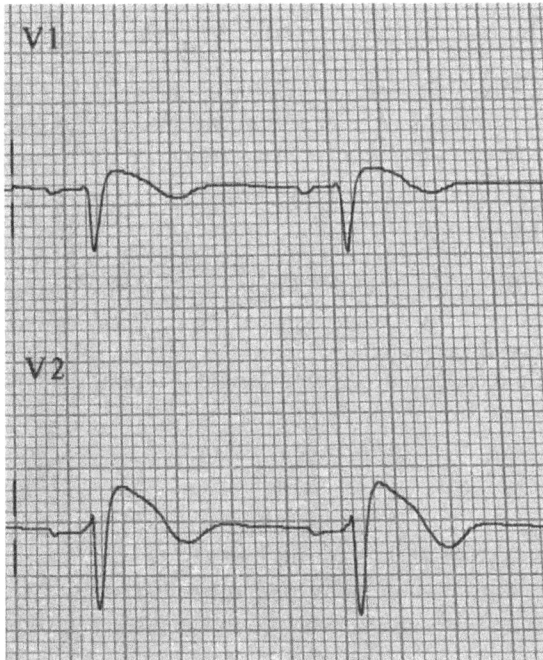

Figure 1. Brugada type 1 pattern.

Several methods can help in case of borderline aspects.

First, refitting the electrodes to the second or third intercostal spaces can reveal a type 1 pattern. Secondly, when type 1 pattern is not spontaneous but it remains a clinical suspicion of Brugada syndrome (e.g., ventricular fibrillation on an apparently healthy heart, unexplained syncope, family history of Brugada syndrome) or an electrocardiographic suspicion (Brugada types 2 and 3 patterns), it is possible to carry out a pharmacological challenge by blocker of the sodium channels to unmask a type 1 pattern [1]. This pharmacological challenge must be carried out in a specialized cardiological environment under strict supervision. Febrile episodes can also unmask a type 1 pattern and increase the risk of ventricular fibrillation.

Around 40% of Brugada syndrome cases are familial forms, thus linked to genetic mutations [3]. With 20–30% of familial forms, mutations of the SCN5A gene are the most common mutations identified. SCN5A gene encodes the cardiac voltage-gated sodium channel (Nav1.5). These proteins ensure the rapid sodium upstroke, resulting in cellular depolarization [4, 5]. Studies of mutations linked to the development of Brugada syndrome revealed loss of Nav1.5 function, thus indicating a decreased amount of sodium going through the cardiomyocyte membrane. The loss of function appears to be shared by all SCN5A mutations but the molecular underlying mechanism can slightly vary from a trafficking defect to alterations in the biophysical properties. While this does not affect the final result, this is an important characteristic that could in the future determine the appropriate pharmacology.

The loss of sodium channel function is expected to cause an imbalance between depolarizing and hyperpolarizing currents in cardiomyocytes. Furthermore, as shown in the next sections, epicardium and endocardium present different levels of repolarizing currents such as Ito currents. This difference would increase the depolarizing/hyperpolarizing imbalance underlying the ST elevation and promote an arrhythmogenic substrate.

The rational to the use of Nav blockers to unmask Brugada ECG phenotypes is thus notably supported by the high occurrence of SNC5A mutations. Consequently, in case of SCN5A mutation, the use of a Nav blocker will rapidly unmask the phenotype. In case where a SCN5A mutation is not involved, larger doses of Nav blocker could mimic a SCN5A mutation and thus reveal the phenotype.

The old types 2 and 3, with saddle-back ST segment elevation, no longer allow to make the diagnosis.

The diagnosis of Brugada syndrome remains context-dependent, as illustrated in the next section.

2.2. Phenocopies

A number of pathological conditions can mimic a Brugada type 1 pattern on the electrocardiogram. The works of Baranchuk and Anselm has improved knowledge in this area [6]. These observations are rare and no large series has allowed studying it yet.

Several clinical cases highlight many underlying conditions. Type 1 Brugada phenocopies have been observed in various cardiac diseases (myocardial ischemia such inferior infarction with right ventricle extension or anterior infarction [7–9], Tako-Tsubo cardiomyopathy [10], cardiac tumors [11], Chagas disease [12]), in pulmonary and mediastinal diseases (acute pulmonary embolism [13], pneumothorax [14], mediastinal tumors [15]), in metabolic and hydroelectrolytic disorders (hypokalemia [16, 17], hyperkalemia [18], hyponatremia [19], hypophosphatemia [20], keto-acidosis [21]), in intoxications (heroin and ethanol overdose [22], propofol [23], propafenone [24], yellow phosphorus [25], lamotrigine [26], phosphine [27]), and various diseases such intracranial hemorrhages [28], hypothermia [29], and electrocution [30]. Pectus excavatum can also mimic a type 1 pattern [31].

According to Baranchuk and Anselm [6], the diagnosis of phenocopy is based on the context, on the normalization of the ECG with the resolution of the cause, and on the negativity of the pharmacological challenge.

The prognostic impact of phenocopies is poorly documented.

3. Electrocardiographic risk markers

3.1. Type 1 pattern

3.1.1. Spontaneous type 1 pattern

The spontaneous nature of the ECG type 1 pattern (contrary to the drug-induced type 1) seems to indicate an increased risk of ventricular fibrillation. This was demonstrated in 2005 by Eckardt et al. [32] and has since been found in several large studies, particularly in the FINGER cohort [33] involving 1029 patients, where a spontaneous type 1 pattern was predictive of a greater risk of sudden death with a hazard ratio (HR) of 1.8 (CI 1.03–3.33, p = 0.04).

A study by Cerrato et al. [34] has shown that the use of the 24-h holter ECG monitoring can help with spontaneous type 1 diagnosis, which is more common during the sleep. This method could be an alternative to avoid the risks related to the pharmacological challenge.

3.1.2. Duration of type 1 pattern expression

Similarly, Extramiana et al. [35] showed by holter ECG monitoring that permanent type 1 expression was associated with an increased risk of syncope and/or ventricular fibrillation.

The 24 or 48 h-holter ECG monitoring could therefore be an interesting tool in the stratification of patients' risk.

Two opposed theories [36] can explain the electrocardiographic and rhythmic abnormalities observed in the Brugada syndrome: a so-called depolarization theory and a so-called repolarization theory. The abnormalities of depolarization and repolarization explain a number of ECG changes that may indicate a poor prognosis.

3.2. Depolarization and conduction disorders

3.2.1. Supraventricular level

3.2.1.1. Sinus node dysfunction

The sinus node dysfunction (**Figure 2**) frequently observed in Brugada syndrome is the conjunction of two phenomena secondary to the reduction of sodium current: an alteration of sinus tissue function and a sino-atrial functional block [37]. Sinus node dysfunction is more frequent in case of mutation on the SCN5A gene [38].

A study conducted on 400 patients by Siera et al. [39] showed that sinus dysfunction was a predictor of ventricular fibrillation risk. The same observation was also made on a cohort of children [40] and a cohort of women [41] with Brugada syndrome (**Table 1**).

3.2.1.2. First degree atrioventricular block

Maury et al. [42] showed in a study of 325 patients with Brugada type 1 that the presence of first-degree atrioventricular block (**Figure 3**) was significantly associated in multivariate analysis with increasing risk of ventricular fibrillation (OR 2.41, 95% CI 1.01–5.73, p = 0.046) (**Table 2**).

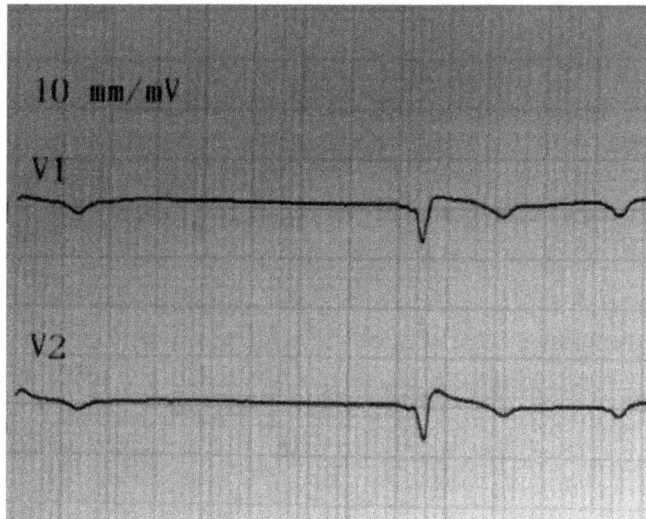

Figure 2. Sinus pause in a 54-year-old woman with Brugada type 1 syndrome and recurrence of syncopes.

- clinical-electrical criterion with correlation between symptoms (faintness, syncope) and a documented event among sinus bradycardia, sinus arrest, sick sinus syndrome, and chronotropic incompetence;
- A Holter ECG was practiced in case of doubt to correlate electrical events and symptoms; and
- electrophysiological exploration of the sinus node was also performed.

Table 1. Criteria of sinus node dysfunction in Sieira et al. study [41].

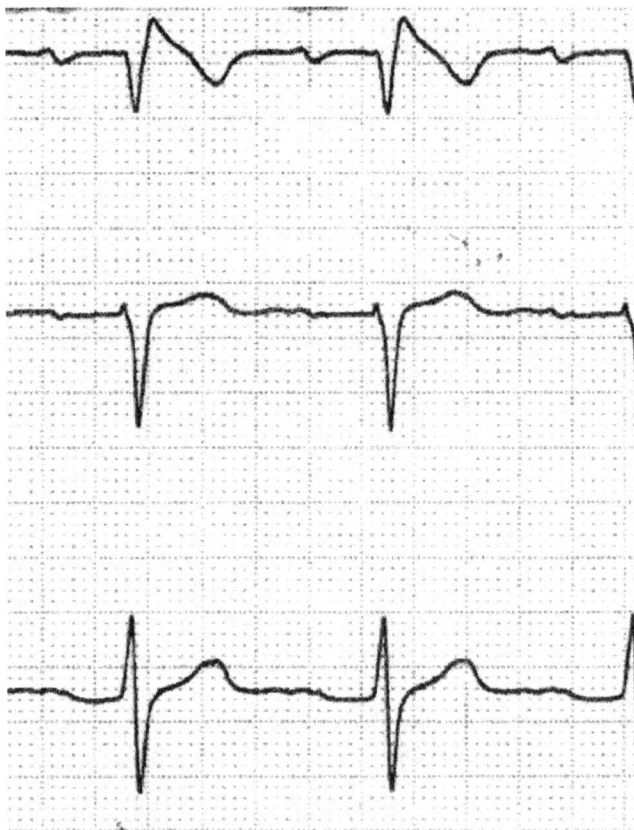

Figure 3. First-degree AVB in a woman with Brugada type 1 pattern.

In addition, Smits et al. [38] demonstrated that atrioventricular conduction abnormalities were significantly increased in the case of SCN5A gene mutation. A PR interval ≥ 210 ms would be a good predictor of a mutation in the SCN5A gene in Brugada syndrome. Previous observations [43, 44] have shown that sodium channels genes mutations are also implicated in conduction disturbances in Lev/Lenegre disease.

3.2.2. Ventricular level

3.2.2.1. Pathophysiology

Cardiac imaging tests (transthoracic echocardiography, angiography, MRI) are usually normal in Brugada syndrome, so it was long believed that this pathology did not lead to heart structural abnormalities. Several recent studies question this dogma.

PR interval ≥ 200 ms

Table 2. First-degree atrioventricular block criterion in Maury et al. study [42].

Functional studies using surface ECG mapping [45], tissular Doppler imaging [46], and endo- and epicardial electrophysiology [47, 48] show that there is an abnormally long conduction delay in the epicardium of the right ventricular outflow tract. This conduction delay is some- times accompanied by late ventricular potentials [48].

Several factors may explain these abnormalities of conduction. On the one hand, the decrease of the incoming sodium current reduces the intramyocardial conduction veloc- ity [49], while on the other hand, histological and histochemical studies [50, 51] reveal the abnormally large presence of fibrosis deposits in the epicardium of the right ventri- cle outflow tract, these deposits are accompanied locally by a reduction in expression of gap-junctions. An experimental model in the mouse showed that these two abnormalities could be the consequence of the decrease of SCN5A gene expression [52].

The shift created between the depolarization (and thereby, secondarily, the repolarization) of the right ventricular outflow tract and the other segments of the ventricles could thus explain the ST segment elevation and the negativity of the T waves [36].

Several studies show that the importance of these conduction abnormalities is highly variable between patients with Brugada syndrome and is correlated with the risk of ventricular fibril- lation [53].

These findings are supported by several interventional studies highlighting the lower recur- rence of ventricular rhythmic events after radiofrequency ablation in the right ventricular outflow tract [54].

It is therefore important to estimate the importance of impairment of right ventricular con- duction in patients to determine their level of risk of sudden death. Several ECG markers can help with a non-invasive evaluation.

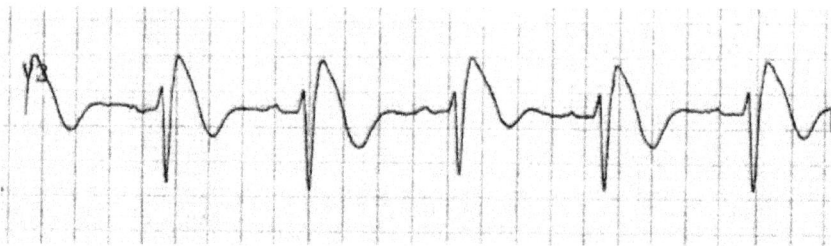

Figure 4. Wide QRS in lead V2 in a patient with a Brugada type 1 pattern.

In lead V2, width of QRS ≥ 120 ms

Table 3. Wide QRS criterion on Ohkubo et al. study [55].

3.2.2.2. Wide QRS in lead V2

Wide QRS in lead V2 (**Figure 4**) is the most obvious marker of alteration of right ventricular conduction. The widening of the QRS in V2 classically demonstrates a slowdown of conduction in the right ventricle.

Ohkubo et al. [55] found, in a cohort of 35 patients with Brugada syndrome, a significant association between wide QRS in lead V2 and ventricular fibrillation and/or syncope (**Table 3**).

3.2.2.3. S-waves in lead DI

Based on the assumption that S-waves in lead DI are the translation of the third vector resulting from the depolarization of right ventricular outflow tract and the basal parts of the two ventricles, Calò et al. [56] demonstrated an electroanatomical correlation between the epicardial activation time of the right ventricular outflow tract and the importance of S-waves in DI.

The same team has shown in a multicentric study [56] of 347 patients with spontaneous type 1, that significant S-waves in lead DI (**Figure 5**) represent a strong marker of risk of sudden death, with a sensitivity of 90.6% and a specificity of 62.2% for the depth of the waves and a sensitivity of 96.9% and a specificity of 61.1% for the duration of the waves (**Table 4**).

The right ventricular outflow tract is notably the last structure responsible to eject the blood to the pulmonary artery. This is notably ensured by a delay in action potentials. While such delay constitutes a physiological need, it also creates a first-degree heterogeneity between this specific structure and the right ventricle. In the background of a SCN5A mutation, such heterogeneity would be even more pronounced, making the right ventricular outflow tract a pro-arrhythmogenic area.

3.2.2.4. The aVR sign

The positivity of the QRS complexes in lead aVR (**Figure 6**) may reflect a right ventricular conduction delay responsible for a right axial deviation of the QRS.

Babai Bigi et al. [57] found in a prospective cohort of 24 patients with a Brugada type 1 pattern a significant association between the presence of significant R-waves in aVR and the risk of syncope and/or ventricular fibrillation (**Table 5**).

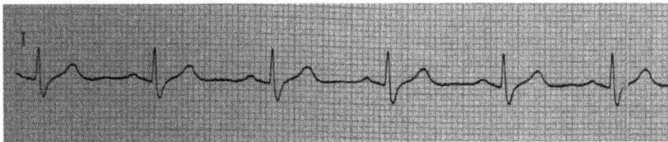

Figure 5. Significant S-waves in lead DI.

In lead DI, S-waves with a depth of at least 0.1 mV and/or a width of at least 40 ms

Table 4. Criteria of S-waves in Calò et al. study [56].

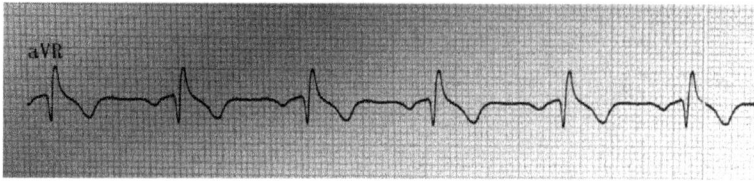

Figure 6. aVR sign.

In lead aVR, R-wave ≥0.3 mV and/or R/q ratio ≥ 0.75

Table 5. Criterion of aVR sign in Babai Bigi et al. study [57].

3.2.2.5. Fragmented QRS

Fragmented QRS (**Figure 7**) were first described in ischemic cardiomyopathies [58], where they are a sign of significant fibrotic scars and lead to a risk of malignant ventricular arrhythmias by macro-reentry. They could also testify of the importance of right ventricular fibrosis in Brugada syndrome. Morita et al. [49] also showed the existence of a dynamic part to this pattern, varying according to the conditions of conduction.

The same team showed [49], with a cohort of 115 patients with Brugada syndrome, that fragment QRS were significantly more frequent in the ventricular fibrillation group (**Table 6**).

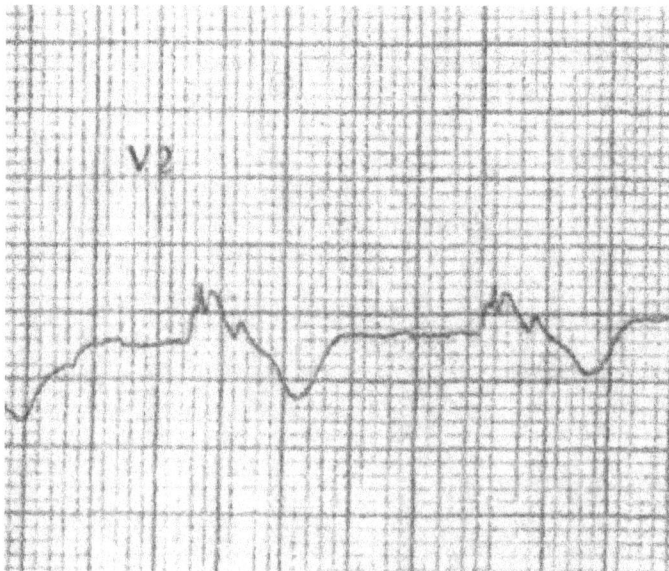

Figure 7. Fragmented QRS in a patient with a Brugada type 1 pattern.

- In leads V1, V2, and V3: ≥4 spikes in a derivation and/or ≥8 spikes in these 3 leads
- The filters must be kept to a minimum so that they do not erase the spikes, especially with a high frequency cut-off (around 150 Hz). This explains why fragmented QRS are often missing on standard ECG.

Table 6. Criteria of fragmented QRS in Morita et al. study [49].

3.3. Repolarization disorders

3.3.1. Pathophysiology

The repolarization theory was mainly developed in the works of Antzelevitch [59–61].

The right ventricular outflow tract epicardial cells hold more I_{to} potassium channels than other myocardial cells. In the Brugada syndrome, the reduction of the sodium current accentuates locally in the right ventricular outflow tract the shortening duration of the action potentials induced by the important activity of the I_{to} channels. A voltage gradient is thus created between the endocardium and the epicardium, resulting in the dome-shaped ST elevation observed on the ECG. Brugada syndrome thus carries a risk of ventricular fibrillation by Phase 2 reentry mechanism.

This theory is usually opposed to the theory of conduction described earlier [62].

3.3.2. Tpeak-Tend interval, QT

The three types of ventricular myocardial cells have different repolarization durations [61]. The epicardial cells are the most rapidly repolarized, then the endocardial cells, and finally the M-cells. Thus, the peak of the T waves corresponds with the moment when the epicardial cells are completely repolarized and the end of the T waves coincides with the end of the repolarization of the M-cells. Therefore, the Tp-e, corresponding with the interval between the vertex and the end of the T waves, is considered by many authors [63] as proportional to the importance of the transmural dispersion of repolarization in the ventricular myocardium. A wide dispersion of repolarization increases myocardial vulnerability and therefore the risk of arrhythmia. An elongated Tp-e would thus translate into a high risk of sudden death by ventricular arrhythmia.

Maury et al. [64] showed in 2015 with a large retrospective cohort of 325 patients, that a maximum Tp-e in precordial leads greater than or equal to 100 ms was significantly and independently associated with an increased risk of ventricular fibrillation in Brugada syndrome (**Table 7**).

Similarly, a study by Castro Hevia et al. [65] highlighted a correlation between a Tpeak-Tend dispersion (difference between Tpeak-Tend maximum and minimum in precordial shunt) > 20 ms and a risk of ventricular fibrillation.

QT interval prolongation may also means a worse prognosis in Brugada syndrome [65].

3.3.3. Early repolarization

Haïssaguerre et al. [66] have recently individualized the early repolarization syndrome, which associates an early repolarization pattern (**Figure 8**) with malignant ventricular

Maximum Tpeak-Tend adjusted to heart rate among leads V1–V4 ≥ 100 ms

Tpeak-Tend measurement method:

- From lead V1 to lead V4
- Measurement of the interval between the peak of the T wave and the tangent between the downward slope of the T wave and the isoelectric line
- Average of three consecutive complexes by derivation
- Correction of the heart rate according to the Bazett method (Tp-e corrected = Tp-e/$\sqrt{RR}$)

Table 7. Criteria of prolonged maximum Tpeak-Tend interval in Maury et al. study [64].

arrhythmia. Antzelevitch and Yan [67] have shown that the pathophysiology of this syndrome is close to the repolarization theory of Brugada syndrome: a large repolarization heterogeneity in the left ventricle could lead to a risk of ventricular fibrillation by Phase 2 reentry. The association of both syndromes would result in repolarization heterogeneity in both the right ventricle and the inferior lateral parts of the left ventricle with a high risk of ventricular fibrillation [67, 68].

Kawata et al. [68] showed, in a cohort of 49 patients with Brugada type 1 syndrome and a history of ventricular fibrillation, that the presence of a permanent early repolarization pattern (HR 4.88, 95% CI 2.02–12.7) or intermittent (HR 2.50, 95% CI 1.03–6.43) was significantly (p = 0.043) associated with a higher risk of recurrence of a fatal rhythmic event (**Table 8**).

3.4. Other electrocardiographic markers

3.4.1. Atrial fibrillation

Calò et al. [56] showed through a multivariate analysis of 347 patients that the occurrence of atrial fibrillation (**Figure 9**) episodes in Brugada type 1 patients was a significant and independent risk marker for ventricular fibrillation.

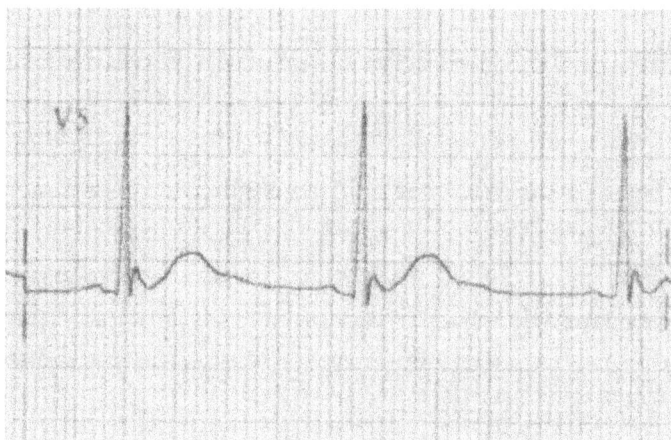

Figure 8. Early repolarization pattern (notching).

J-point elevation at least 1 mm in at least two inferior or lateral leads (either notching or slurring pattern)

Table 8. Early repolarization criteria in Kawata et al. study [68].

In at least one peripheral derivation (aVR included):
- coved ST segment elevation with J-point rise ≥2 mm
- and negative T waves in the same derivation.

Table 9. Criteria of type 1 in peripheral lead pattern in Rollin et al. study [69].

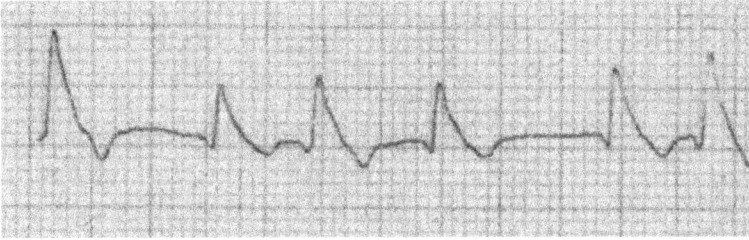

Figure 9. Atrial fibrillation in a patient with Brugada type 1 pattern.

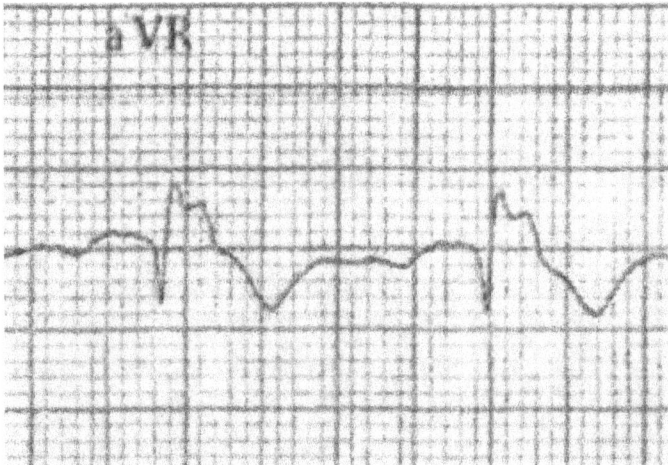

Figure 10. Type 1 pattern in peripheral lead (aVR).

3.4.2. Type 1 in peripheral leads

In a study by Rollin et al. [69] conducted on 323 patients, a type 1 pattern in peripheral leads (**Figure 10**) appears to be an independent marker of high risk of ventricular fibrillation (**Table 9**). In total, 27% of patients with type 1 in peripheral leads showed malignant ventricular arrhythmia, compared to 6% for other patients. The multivariate analysis confirms a strong correlation (OR 4.58, 95% CI 1.7–12.32, p = 0.025).

The pathophysiological significance of this aspect still needs to be clarified.

4. Conclusion

The surface electrocardiogram is the key examination in Brugada syndrome. It is currently the only means to allow diagnosis and it could help stratification of the ventricular fibrillation risk. In the last few years, numerous publications highlighted several electrocardiographic markers testifying to a more severe disease and a potentially unfavorable prognosis. These markers also contributed to the improvement of knowledge of the physiopathology of this syndrome. However, studies are still needed to determine their use in daily practice.

Author details

Antoine Deliniere, Francis Bessiere, Adrien Moreau, Alexandre Janin, Gilles Millat and Philippe Chevalier*

*Address all correspondence to: philippe.chevalier@chu-lyon.fr

Hôpital Louis Pradel, Lyon, France

References

[1] Priori SG, Blomström-Lundqvist C, Mazzanti A, Blom N, Borggrefe M, Camm J, et al. 2015 ESC Guidelines for the management of patients with ventricular arrhythmias and the prevention of sudden cardiac death The Task Force for the Management of Patients with Ventricular Arrhythmias and the Prevention of Sudden Cardiac Death of the European Society of Cardiology (ESC) Endorsed by: Association for European Paediatric and Congenital Cardiology (AEPC). European Heart Journal. 2015;**36**(41):2793-2867

[2] Sieira J, Brugada P. The definition of the Brugada syndrome. European Heart Journal. 2017;**38**(40):3029-3034

[3] Watanabe H, Minamino T. Genetics of Brugada syndrome. Journal of Human Genetics. 2016;**61**(1):57-60

[4] Amin AS, Tan HL, Wilde AAM. Cardiac ion channels in health and disease. Heart Rhythm. 2010;**7**(1):117-126

[5] Ruan Y, Liu N, Priori SG. Sodium channel mutations and arrhythmias. Nature Reviews. Cardiology. 2009;**6**(5):337-348

[6] Anselm DD, Evans JM, Baranchuk A. Brugada phenocopy: A new electrocardiogram phenomenon. World Journal of Cardiology. 2014;**6**(3):81-86

[7]   Agrawal S, Stevens S, Shirani J, Garg J, Nanda S. Ischemia-induced Brugada phenocopy. Journal of Electrocardiology. 2015;**48**(5):815-817

[8]   Gottschalk BH, Anselm DD, Baranchuk A. Coronary anomalies resulting in ischemia induced Brugada Phenocopy. International Journal of Cardiology. 2015;**199**:75-76

[9]   Ferrando-Castagnetto F, Garibaldi-Remuñan A, Vignolo G, Ricca-Mallada R, Baranchuk A. Brugada phenocopy as a dynamic electrocardiographic pattern during acute anterior myocardial infarction. Annals of Noninvasive Electrocardiology: The Official Journal of the International Society for Holter and Noninvasive Electrocardiology, Inc. 2016;**21**(4):425-428

[10] Kirbas O, Ozeke O, Karabulut O, Unal S, Sen F, Cagli K, et al. Warm-up Brugada phenocopy associated with takotsubo cardiomyopathy. American Journal of Emergency Medicine. 2016;**34**(10):2051.e1-2051.e3

[11] Nguyen T, Smythe J, Baranchuk A. Rhabdomyoma of the interventricular septum presenting as a Brugada phenocopy. Cardiology in the Young. 2011;**21**(5):591-594

[12] Arce M, Riera ARP, Femenía F, Baranchuk A. Brugada electrocardiographic phenocopy in a patient with chronic Chagasic cardiomyopathy. Cardiology Journal. 2010;**17**(5):525-527

[13] Zhan Z-Q, Wang C-Q, Nikus KC, Pérez-Riera AR, Baranchuk A. Brugada phenocopy in acute pulmonary embolism. International Journal of Cardiology. 2014;**177**(3):e153-e155

[14] Barcos JC, Tello IS, Monié CC, Fernández MR, Humphreys JD. Brugada phenocopy induced by severe pneumothorax. Journal of Electrocardiology. 2018;**51**(2):343-345

[15] Tarín N, Farré J, Rubio JM, Tuñón J, Castro-Dorticós J. Brugada-like electrocardiographic pattern in a patient with a mediastinal tumor. Pacing and Clinical Electrophysiology. 1999;**22**(8):1264-1266

[16] Genaro NR, Anselm DD, Cervino N, Estevez AO, Perona C, Villamil AM, et al. Brugada phenocopy clinical reproducibility demonstrated by recurrent hypokalemia. Annals of Noninvasive Electrocardiology: The Official Journal of the International Society for Holter and Noninvasive Electrocardiology, Inc. 2014;**19**(4):387-390

[17] Anselm DD, Genaro NR, Baranchuk A. Possible brugada phenocopy induced by hypokalemia in a patient with congenital hypokalemic periodic paralysis. Arquivos Brasileiros de Cardiologia. 2014;**102**(1):104

[18] Abu Shama R, Bayes de Luna A, Baranchuk A. Tachycardia-dependent Brugada phenocopy due to hyperkalemia. Journal of Cardiovascular Electrophysiology. 2017; **28**(9):1084-1085

[19] Agrawal Y, Aggarwal S, Kalavakunta JK, Gupta V. All that looks like "Brugada" is not "Brugada": Case series of Brugada phenocopy caused by hyponatremia. Journal of the Saudi Heart Association. 2016;**28**(4):274-277

[20] Meloche J, Gottschalk BH, Boles U, LaHaye S, Baranchuk A. Hypophosphatemia as a novel etiology of Brugada Phenocopy. International Journal of Cardiology. 2016;**208**:70-71

[21] Alanzalon RE, Burris JR, Vinocur JM. Brugada phenocopy associated with diabetic keto-
      acidosis in two pediatric patients. Journal of Electrocardiology. 2018 Mar 1;**51**(2):323-326

[22] Rambod M, Elhanafi S, Mukherjee D. Brugada phenocopy in concomitant ethanol and
      heroin overdose. Annals of Noninvasive Electrocardiology: The Official Journal of the
      International Society for Holter and Noninvasive Electrocardiology, Inc. 2015;**20**(1):87-90

[23] Riera ARP, Uchida AH, Schapachnik E, Dubner S, Filho CF, Ferreira C. Propofol infu-
      sion syndrome and Brugada syndrome electrocardiographic phenocopy. Cardiology
      Journal. 2010;**17**(2):130-135

[24] Arı ME, Ekici F. Brugada-phenocopy induced by propafenone overdose and successful
      treatment: A case report. Balkan Medical Journal. 2017;**34**(5):473-475

[25] Dharanipradab M, Viswanathan S, Kumar GR, Krishnamurthy V, Stanley DD. Yellow
      phosphorus-induced Brugada phenocopy. Journal of Electrocardiology. 2018;**51**(1):
      129-131

[26] Rodrigues R, Amador P, Rassi L, Seixo F, Parreira L, Fonseca N, et al. Brugada pat-
      tern in a patient medicated with lamotrigine. Revista Portuguesa de Cardiologia: Orgão
      Oficial da Sociedade Portuguesa de Cardiologia = Portuguese Journal of Cardiology: An
      Official Journal of the Portuguese Society of Cardiology. 2013;**32**(10):807-810

[27] Gottschalk BH, Anselm DD, Baranchuk A. Phosphine poisoning is emerging as an
      important cause of Brugada Phenocopy. Pacing and Clinical Electrophysiology. 2016;
      39(2):202-203

[28] Labadet C, Gottschalk BH, Rivero M, Hadid C, Fuselli J, Anselm DD, et al. Brugada phe-
      nocopy in the context of intracranial hemorrhage. International Journal of Cardiology.
      2014;**177**(3):e156-e157

[29] Gottschalk B, Anselm DD, Baranchuk A. Suspected Brugada phenocopy in the context of
      hypothermia. Acta Cardiologica. 2014;**69**(4):454-455

[30] Wang JG, McIntyre WF, Kong W, Baranchuk A. Electrocution-induced Brugada pheno-
      copy. International Journal of Cardiology. 2012;**160**(3):e35-e37

[31] Awad SFM, Barbosa-Barros R, Belem L de S, Cavalcante CP, Riera ARP, Garcia-Niebla
      J, et al. Brugada phenocopy in a patient with pectus excavatum: Systematic review of
      the ECG manifestations associated with pectus excavatum. Annals of Noninvasive
      Electrocardiology: The Official Journal of the International Society for Holter and
      Noninvasive Electrocardiology, Inc. 2013;**18**(5):415-20

[32] Eckardt L, Probst V, Smits JPP, Bahr ES, Wolpert C, Schimpf R, et al. Long-term prog-
      nosis of individuals with right precordial ST-segment-elevation Brugada syndrome.
      Circulation. 2005;**111**(3):257-263

[33] Probst V, Veltmann C, Eckardt L, Meregalli PG, Gaita F, Tan HL, et al. Long-term prog-
      nosis of patients diagnosed with Brugada syndrome: Results from the FINGER Brugada
      Syndrome Registry. Circulation. 2010;**121**(5):635-643

[34] Cerrato N, Giustetto C, Gribaudo E, Richiardi E, Barbonaglia L, Scrocco C, et al. Prevalence of type 1 brugada electrocardiographic pattern evaluated by twelve-lead twenty-four-hour holter monitoring. The American Journal of Cardiology. 2015;**115**(1):52-56

[35] Extramiana F, Maison-Blanche P, Badilini F, Messali A, Denjoy I, Leenhardt A. Type 1 electrocardiographic burden is increased in symptomatic patients with Brugada syndrome. Journal of Electrocardiology. 2010;**43**(5):408-414

[36] Meregalli PG, Wilde AAM, Tan HL. Pathophysiological mechanisms of Brugada syndrome: Depolarization disorder, repolarization disorder, or more? Cardiovascular Research. 2005;**67**(3):367-378

[37] Morita H, Fukushima-Kusano K, Nagase S, Miyaji K, Hiramatsu S, Banba K, et al. Sinus node function in patients with Brugada-type ECG. Circulation Journal is the official journal of the Japanese Circulation Society. 2004;**68**(5):473-476

[38] Smits JPP, Eckardt L, Probst V, Bezzina CR, Schott JJ, Remme CA, et al. Genotype-phenotype relationship in Brugada syndrome: Electrocardiographic features differentiate SCN5A-related patients from non-SCN5A-related patients. Journal of the American College of Cardiology. 2002;**40**(2):350-356

[39] Sieira J, Conte G, Ciconte G, Chierchia G-B, Casado-Arroyo R, Baltogiannis G, et al. A score model to predict risk of events in patients with Brugada Syndrome. European Heart Journal. 2017;**38**(22):1756-1763

[40] Gonzalez Corcia MC, Sieira J, Pappaert G, de Asmundis C, Chierchia GB, Sarkozy A, et al. A clinical score model to predict lethal events in young patients (≤19 years) with the Brugada syndrome. The American Journal of Cardiology. 2017;**120**(5):797-802

[41] Sieira J, Conte G, Ciconte G, de Asmundis C, Chierchia G-B, Baltogiannis G, et al. Clinical characterisation and long-term prognosis of women with Brugada syndrome. Heart (British Cardiac Society). 2016;**102**(6):452-458

[42] Maury P, Rollin A, Sacher F, Gourraud J-B, Raczka F, Pasquié J-L, et al. Prevalence and prognostic role of various conduction disturbances in patients with the Brugada syndrome. The American Journal of Cardiology. 2013;**112**(9):1384-1389

[43] Schott JJ, Alshinawi C, Kyndt F, Probst V, Hoorntje TM, Hulsbeek M, et al. Cardiac conduction defects associate with mutations in SCN5A. Nature Genetics. 1999;**23**(1):20-21

[44] Tan HL, Bink-Boelkens MT, Bezzina CR, Viswanathan PC, Beaufort-Krol GC, van Tintelen PJ, et al. A sodium-channel mutation causes isolated cardiac conduction disease. Nature. 2001;**409**(6823):1043-1047

[45] Postema PG, van Dessel PFHM, de Bakker JMT, Dekker LRC, Linnenbank AC, Hoogendijk MG, et al. Slow and discontinuous conduction conspire in Brugada syndrome: A right ventricular mapping and stimulation study. Circulation. Arrhythmia and Electrophysiology. 2008;**1**(5):379-386

[46] Van Malderen SCH, Kerkhove D, Theuns DAMJ, Weytjens C, Droogmans S, Tanaka K, et al. Prolonged right ventricular ejection delay identifies high risk patients and gender differences in Brugada syndrome. International Journal of Cardiology. 2015;**191**:90-96

[47] Lambiase PD, Ahmed AK, Ciaccio EJ, Brugada R, Lizotte E, Chaubey S, et al. High-density substrate mapping in Brugada syndrome: Combined role of conduction and repolarization heterogeneities in Arrhythmogenesis. Circulation. 2009;**120**(2):106-117

[48] Nagase S, Kusano KF, Morita H, Fujimoto Y, Kakishita M, Nakamura K, et al. Epicardial electrogram of the right ventricular outflow tract in patients with the brugada syndrome: Using the epicardial lead. Journal of the American College of Cardiology. 2002; **39**(12):1992-1995

[49] Morita H, Kusano KF, Miura D, Nagase S, Nakamura K, Morita ST, et al. Fragmented QRS as a marker of conduction abnormality and a predictor of prognosis of Brugada syndrome. Circulation. 2008;**118**(17):1697-1704

[50] Coronel R, Casini S, Koopmann TT, Wilms-Schopman FJG, Verkerk AO, de Groot JR, et al. Right ventricular fibrosis and conduction delay in a patient with clinical signs of Brugada syndrome: A combined electrophysiological, genetic, histopathologic, and computational study. Circulation. 2005;**112**(18):2769-2777

[51] Nademanee K, Raju H, de Noronha SV, Papadakis M, Robinson L, Rothery S, et al. Fibrosis, Connexin-43, and conduction abnormalities in the Brugada syndrome. Journal of the American College of Cardiology. 2015;**66**(18):1976-1986

[52] van Veen TAB, Stein M, Royer A, Quang KL, Charpentier F, Colledge WH, et al. Impaired impulse propagation in Scn5a-knockout mice: Combined contribution of excitability, Connexin expression, and tissue architecture in relation to aging. Circulation. 2005; **112**(13):1927-1935

[53] Doi A, Takagi M, Maeda K, Tatsumi H, Shimeno K, Yoshiyama M. Conduction delay in right ventricle as a marker for identifying high-risk patients with Brugada syndrome. Journal of Cardiovascular Electrophysiology. 2010;**21**(6):688-696

[54] Nademanee K, Veerakul G, Chandanamattha P, Chaothawee L, Ariyachaipanich A, Jirasirirojanakorn K, et al. Prevention of ventricular fibrillation episodes in Brugada syndrome by catheter ablation over the anterior right ventricular outflow tract EpicardiumClinical perspective. Circulation. 2011;**123**(12):1270-1279

[55] Ohkubo K, Watanabe I, Okumura Y, Ashino S, Kofune M, Nagashima K, et al. Prolonged QRS duration in lead V2 and risk of life-threatening ventricular arrhythmia in patients with Brugada syndrome. International Heart Journal. 2011;**52**(2):98-102

[56] Calò L, Giustetto C, Martino A, Sciarra L, Cerrato N, Marziali M, et al. A new electrocardiographic marker of sudden death in Brugada syndrome: The S-wave in lead I. Journal of the American College of Cardiology. 2016;**67**(12):1427-1440

[57] Babai Bigi MA, Aslani A, Shahrzad S. aVR sign as a risk factor for life-threatening arrhythmic events in patients with Brugada syndrome. Heart Rhythm. 2007;**4**(8):1009-1012

[58] Das MK, Saha C, El Masry H, Peng J, Dandamudi G, Mahenthiran J, et al. Fragmented QRS on a 12-lead ECG: A predictor of mortality and cardiac events in patients with coronary artery disease. Heart Rhythm. 2007;**4**(11):1385-1392

[59] Antzelevitch C. The Brugada syndrome. Journal of Cardiovascular Electrophysiology. 1998;**9**(5):513-516

[60] Antzelevitch C. Genetic, molecular and cellular mechanisms underlying the J wave syndromes. Circulation Journal is the official journal of the Japanese Circulation Society. 2012;**76**(5):1054-1065

[61] Antzelevitch C, Dumaine R. Electrical Heterogeneity in the Heart: Physiological, Pharhmacological and Clinical Implications. In: Comprehensive Physiology [Internet]. John Wiley & Sons, Inc.; 2011 [cited 2017 Dec 31]. Available from: http://onlinelibrary.wiley.com/doi/10.1002/cphy.cp020117/abstract

[62] Veerakul G, Nademanee K. Brugada syndrome: Two decades of progress. Circulation Journal is the official journal of the Japanese Circulation Society. 2012;**76**(12):2713-2722

[63] Tse G, Gong M, Wong WT, Georgopoulos S, Letsas KP, Vassiliou VS, et al. The Tpeak-tend interval as an electrocardiographic risk marker of arrhythmic and mortality outcomes: A systematic review and meta-analysis. Heart Rhythm. 2017;**14**(8):1131-1137

[64] Maury P, Sacher F, Gourraud J-B, Pasquié J-L, Raczka F, Bongard V, et al. Increased Tpeak-tend interval is highly and independently related to arrhythmic events in Brugada syndrome. Heart Rhythm. 2015;**12**(12):2469-2476

[65] Castro Hevia J, Antzelevitch C, Tornés Bárzaga F, Dorantes Sánchez M, Dorticós Balea F, Zayas Molina R, et al. Tpeak-tend and Tpeak-tend dispersion as risk factors for ventricular tachycardia/ventricular fibrillation in patients with the Brugada syndrome. Journal of the American College of Cardiology. 2006;**47**(9):1828-1834

[66] Haïssaguerre M, Derval N, Sacher F, Jesel L, Deisenhofer I, de Roy L, et al. Sudden cardiac arrest associated with early repolarization. The New England Journal of Medicine. 2008;**358**(19):2016-2023

[67] Antzelevitch C, Yan G-X. J wave syndromes. Heart Rhythm. 2010;**7**(4):549-558

[68] Kawata H, Morita H, Yamada Y, Noda T, Satomi K, Aiba T, et al. Prognostic significance of early repolarization in inferolateral leads in Brugada patients with documented ventricular fibrillation: A novel risk factor for Brugada syndrome with ventricular fibrillation. Heart Rhythm. 2013;**10**(8):1161-1168

[69] Rollin A, Sacher F, Gourraud JB, Pasquié JL, Raczka F, Duparc A, et al. Prevalence, characteristics, and prognosis role of type 1 ST elevation in the peripheral ECG leads in patients with Brugada syndrome. Heart Rhythm. 2013;**10**(7):1012-1018

Gene Polymorphisms Associated with Atrial Fibrillation

Nevra Alkanli, Arzu Ay and Suleyman Serdar Alkanli

Abstract

Atrial fibrillation (AF), which causes severe health problems, is a multi-factor disorder and is increasing day by day. AF is known to be one of the most common cardiac arrhythmias in clinical practice. AF can also be described as a cardiac dysrhythmia that causes severe cardiovascular morbidity and mortality. AF is known as an independent risk factor for death and it occurs a significant risk of morbidity due to stroke. There are many diseases that contribute to the development of AF. Diseases such as aging, heart failure, heart valve disorders, myocardial infarction, hypertension and diabetes mellitus are important factors in the development of structural AF. It is a known fact that AF prevalence increases with age. The mechanism underlying of AF is not fully understood, but genetic factors play an important role in the pathogenesis of this disease. There have been many studies aimed at investigating the genetic basis of AF, especially in recent years. In these studies, many mutations and variants have emerged which are identified as genetic risk factors in the development of AF. Identification of gene polymorphisms that play a role in the development of AF will be an important guide in the development of new therapies for the treatment of this condition.

Keywords: AF, cardiac arrhythmia, gene polymorphism, related diseases, PCR

1. Introduction

AF, which has a significant morbidity and mortality rate, is a multifactorial disorder as one of the most common cardiac arrhythmias [1, 2]. This cardiac arrhythmia affects 1–2% of the general population. AF is an increasingly prevalent dysrhythmia and is associated with many cardiac risk factors. Disorders such as hypertensive, ischemic or structural heart diseases are important risk factors for AF [3].

The underlying mechanisms in the development of AF are still not fully understood, but a heterogeneous model plays an important role in the pathophysiology of this disease. This heterogeneous model is based on the interaction of multiple substrates and triggers [3].

There are many studies showing that genetic factors play an important role in the pathogenesis of AF. Monogenic mutations known to be associated with AF have been identified. A total of 25 gene mutations proven to be associated with AF have been identified. Genome-wide association studies (GWAS) have been conducted to investigate AF genetics, and these studies have shown that single nucleotide polymorphisms play a very important role in the development of AF. Several single nucleotide polymorphisms associated with AF predisposition have been identified in these GWAS studies [3].

AF is an electrical disease caused by defects in ionic currents, and a variety of studies have been undertaken to determine the genetic causes of these electrical illnesses. Studies conducted to investigate the hereditary predisposition of AF found that the development of AF in pups with AF detected in their parents was found. Even though disorders such as hypertension, myocardial infarction and diabetes mellitus, which are important risk factors for the development of AF, are regulated, they still have the risk of developing fourfold AF [3].

In many genetic studies, variants known to be associated with AF have emerged. These variants are formed as a result of abnormalities in genes encoding cardiac gap junctions, signaling molecules, ion channels and auxiliary subunits. In addition, gene polymorphisms may cause loss of function in genes that encode proteins contributing to cardiac depolarization or repolarization leading to AF's increased sensitivity, are also genetic risk factors that play an important role in the development of AF [3].

The purpose of this chapter is to give general information about AF and compiling the studies made with the aim of determining the gene polymorphisms that can play an important role in the development of AF.

2. Renin angiotensin aldosterone gene polymorphism

The renin angiotensin aldosterone system (RAAS) plays an important role in the regulation of humoral regulation. RAAS, which is also important in the regulation of blood pressure, cardiovascular homeostasis, fluid and electrolyte balance such as hypertension, heart failure and arrhythmia, plays an important role in the pathophysiology of various cardiovascular diseases. Renin, an acid protease synthesized by renal juxtaglomerular cells, is involved in circulation through the renal vein. A decrease in renal blood flow or a decrease in plasma sodium levels leads to an increase in renin secretion. Renin plays a key role in the production of angiotensin I in plasma or tissues. It is provided that renin is converted to angiotensin II by angiotensin-converting enzyme (ACE). Angiotensinogen (AGT), the original subtype of renin, is an important source of angiotensin II. Angiotensin II functions by binding to the angiotensin II receptor on fibroblasts. Angiotensin II plays an important role in enhancing the synthesis and secretion of collagen types I and III in the regulation of proliferation of fibroblasts. Angiotensin II induces aldosterone release, resulting in myocyte necrosis and susceptible fibrosis. RAAS is functioning via angiotensin II. Angiotensin II is involved in the elevation of blood pressure in the systemic arterial and venous systems and in the increase of blood return to the heart. It increases the central sympathetic activity by increasing the oscillation from the sympathetic nerve endings. Thus, synthesis and release of aldosterone is regulated. RAAS, which plays a role in atrial remodeling and pathogenesis of AF, is an important regulator. There are not many studies aiming to investigate the relationship between RAAS gene polymorphisms and the risk of developing AF. In a study conducted by Tsai et al., it was determined that the polymorphisms occurring in RAAS genes increased the susceptibility to AF development as a result of association with environmental factors leading to elevated atrial pressures. RAAS gene polymorphisms include ACE insertion/deletion (I/D), AGT (G-217A, A-20C, G-7A, M235T and T174M) and ATR1 A1166C gene polymorphisms. In a study aiming to investigate the association of these polymorphisms with AF, in exon 2 of the AGT gene, the M235 allele, a significant relationship was found between haploids associated with the G-6 and G-217 alleles in the promoter region and AF development risk [4, 5].

2.1. ACE (I/D) gene polymorphism

The 21-kilobase pair (kbp) long ACE gene locates on chromosome 17q23. This gene consists of 26 exons and 25 introns. The ACE (I/D) gene polymorphism is characterized by I/D of 287 base pairs in the 16th intron of the ACE gene. The genotypes of ACE (I/D) gene polymorphism differ in terms of ACE plasma and tissue levels. The DD genotype of the ACE (I/D) gene polymorphism is associated with high cellular ACE activity, which leads to myocardial fibrosis, so myocardial fibrosis develops. There are studies showing that ACE (I/D) gene polymorphism is associated with the risk of developing AF. There is a positive relationship between DD genotype and ACE activity of ACE (I/D) gene polymorphism. As a result of this relationship, angiotensin II level increases and myocardial hypertrophy, arrhythmia can develop. In the study carried out by Zhang and colleagues found a significant association between DD genotype of the ACE (I/D) gene polymorphism and increased AF. In another study conducted by Topal et al., a significant relationship was found between the incidence of ACE Alu D and increased AF [2].

2.2. ACE 2350G/A (rs4343) gene polymorphism

One of the ACE gene polymorphisms from the AF associated genes is the ACE 2350G/A (rs4343) polymorphism, and this polymorphism has a significant effect on the plasma ACE concentration. The ACE 2350G/A (rs4343) gene polymorphism is a synonymous mutation that is accepted as silent. There is insufficient study to investigate the relationship between ACE 2350G/A (rs4343) gene polymorphism and the risk of developing AF. In a study conducted by Jiang et al. in a Chinese population, the A allele of ACE 2350G/A (rs4343) gene polymorphism has been associated with the risk of developing AF in patients with essential hypertension. ACE 2350G/A (rs4343) polymorphic locus do not effect expression directly of ACE mRNA or it has not functional variant. It is assumed that there may be link imbalance between this fragment and an unknown DNA fragment acting as a muffler. In order to be able to identify gene loci in this linkage disequilibrium, a large number of studies have to be performed [1].

2.3. Angiotensin II type 1 receptor and angiotensin-converting enzyme 2 gene polymorphisms

RAAS, which plays an important role in the pathophysiology of AF in the structural and electrical remodeling of the atrium, contains ACE/angiotensin II/AGTR1 and ACE2/ angiotensin (1–7)/ MAS axes. These axes regulate myocardial hypertrophy, fibrosis and remodeling. ACE/angiotensin II/AGTR1 and ACE2/angiotensin (1–7)/MAS axes have been found to play an important role in AF pathogenesis. Angiotensin II is the most vasoactive component of RAAS, and angiotensin II, which causes increased myocardial fibrosis and hypertrophy, may contribute to AF development. Angiotensin II, an important signaling molecule of RAAS, plays a role in cardiovascular effects via AGTR1. AGTR1, G-protein is a bound receptor and has been associated with some disorders such as heart failure, prehypertension and stroke. There are studies showing that in AF patients AGTR1 levels increase in the left atrium. In a study conducted with Chinese Han population, the roles of AGTR1 rs1492100, rs1492099, rs1492097 and rs3772616 gene polymorphisms in AF development were investigated. A significant correlation was found between rs1492099 gene polymorphism from these polymorphisms and the development of structural AF. The ACE2 gene shows the X chromosome. In a study conducted by Freg et al., ACE2 expression was found to be significantly reduced in patients with chronic AF. In contrast, it is observed that atrial tissue angiotensin II levels were also significantly elevated. In another study with Chinese Han population, the effects of AGTR1 and ACE2 gene polymorphisms development of structural AF were examined. It is thought that polymorphisms occurred in this gene may be genetic risk factors in the development of structural AF in the Chinese Han male population. Also, it has been shown that ACE2 and AGTR1 genes are associated in patients with structural AF [6].

2.4. Aldosterone synthase 344 C/T gene polymorphism

Aldosterone synthase (CYP112B2) is an enzyme that plays an important role in the synthesis of aldosterone. CYP112B2 is the mitochondrial P450 oxidase found in the adrenal cortex of the zona glomerulosa. Aldosterone plays an important role in regulation of ion motions and collagen expression, including myocardial remodeling. Delayed or reversed myocardial remodeling is achieved by the aldosterone inhibitor, thus can prevent AF. In a study by Goette et al., there was a positive relationship between elevation of AF and aldosterone levels. The CYP112B2 gene is 7 kilobases long and locates on chromosome 8q22. This gene consists of 9 exons and 8 introns. The CYP112B2-344 C/T gene polymorphism is characterized by a C/T substitution in the −344 position in the promoter region of the CYP112B2 gene. Several studies have been conducted to investigate the relationship between CYP112B2-344 C/T gene polymorphism and hypertension. In some studies, CYP112B2-344 C/T gene polymorphism has been identified as a genetic risk factor for hypertension and myocardial hypertrophy. However, a limited number of studies have been conducted to investigate the relationship between CYP112B2-344 C/T gene polymorphism and AF. In a study conducted by Lu et al., no significant relationship was found between CYP112B2-344 C/T gene polymorphism and AF development risk. In the study conducted by Shuxin Hou et al., there were no significant differences in CYP112B2-344 C/T gene polymorphism genotype distributions between AF patients and healthy control groups. The CYP112B2-344 C/T gene polymorphism has been

AGTR1 and ACE2	Forward primer 5′-3′	Reverse primer 3′–5′
rs1492100	TTCAATAACAGATTCCCAGAG	CCACCTCAACTTGCCTGTG
rs1492099	TTCAATAACAGATTCCCAGAG	CCACCTCAACTTGCCTGTG
rs1492097	TTCAATAACAGATTCCCAGAG	CCACCTCAACTTGCCTGTG
rs3772616	TGATAATTTATGTACTCCCTC	CAAAGCATAAGTGTCAACAGA
rs6632677	CTGACTTGTTGCAGCAAGATGC	TAGGAGTCCAGGCACAGTTCAG

PCR, polymerase chain reaction; SNP, single nucleotide polymorphism; AGTR1, angiotensin II receptor 1; ACE2, angiotensin-converting enzyme 2; Amp, amplification.

Table 1. Primer sequences used in PCR for AGTR1 and ACE2.

GENES amp. size (bp)	Primer	Primer sequences
AGT M235T 163 bp	Forward	5′-CGTTTGTGCAGGGCCTGGCTCTC-3′
	Reverse	5′-AGGGTGCTGTCCACACTGGACCC-3′
ACE AluI/D 490 bp	Forward	5′-CTGGAGACCACTCCCATCCTTTCT-3′
	Reverse	5′-GATGTGGCCATCACATTCGTCAGAT-3′
CYP112B2-344C/T 537 bp	Forward	5′-CAGGAGGAGACCCCATGTGAC-3′
	Reverse	5′-CCTCCACCCTGTTCAGCC-3′

PCR, polymerase chain reaction; AGT, angiotensinogen; ACE (I/D), angiotensin-converting enzyme (insertion/deletion); CYP112B2, aldosterone synthase; Amp, amplification.

Table 2. Primer sequences used in PCR and amplification product size for AGT, ACE (I/D) and CYP112B2-344C/T.

found to be associated with an increase in C allele binding to steroidogenic transcription factor 1 and thus an increase in CYP112B2 activity. In a study conducted by Amir et al., CYP112B2-344 C/T gene polymorphism CC genotype was found to be an independent risk factor for AF in patients with heart failure. In a study in China Han population, conducted by Huang et al., found that CYP112B2-344 C/T gene polymorphism is not a genetic risk factor in the development of AF in patients with hypertensive heart disease. In a study performed by Zhang et al., the significant relationship is not also found between CYP112B2-344 C/T gene polymorphism and AF development [2]. It is presented primer sequences that used to determine AGTR1, ACE2, AGT, ACE (I/D) and CYP112B2-344C/T gene polymorphisms in **Tables 1** and **2**.

3. Nitric oxide synthase gene polymorphisms

The major products of cellular metabolism are reactive oxygen species (ROS) and reactive nitrogen products (RNS) and they have sources in the myocardium. Redox homeostasis is disturbed when oxidant species overcome the capacity to reduce of the cell. While excessive ROS results in oxidative stress; excessive RNS results in nitrosative stress. Potentially reactive species such as the mitochondrial electron transport chain, xanthine oxidase, NADPH oxidases and nitric oxide synthases (NOS) are present in the myocardium. There are three NOS isoforms: NOS1 (neuronal NOS = nNOS), NOS2 (inducible NOS = iNOS) and NOS3 (endothelial NOS = eNOS). These isoforms are named according to the first description of the tissues. It

Genes amp. size (bp)	Primer	Primer sequences
eNOS T-786 180 bp	Sense	5'-TGGAGAGTGCTGGTGTACCCCA-3'
	Antisense	5'-GCCTCCACCCCACCCTGTC-3'
eNOS G894T 200 bp	Sense	5'-AACCCCCTCTGGCCCACTCCC-3'
	Antisense	5'-TCCATCCCACCCAGTCAA-3'
Intron 4a/4b 393 (4a) 420 (4b)	Sense	5'-AGGCCCTATGGTAGTGCCTTT-3'
	Antisense	5'-TCTCTTAGTGCTGTGGTCAC-3'

PCR, polymerase chain reaction; eNOS, endothelial nitric oxide synthase; Amp, amplification.

Table 3. Sequence of primers, size of the PCR products eNOS T-786C, G894T, Intron 4a/4b gene polymorphisms.

is known that enzymes that occur in NOS1 and NOS3 are expressed in the heart. NOS2 is expressed in inflammatory and pathological conditions such as hypertrophy or heart failure. While in cardiac myocytes, NOS1 and NOS3 were present in intracellular compartments, NOS2 is present in the cytosol of cardiac myocytes. NOS plays an important role in stimulating effects of NO on guanylate cyclase, or in arising and mediating effects of nitrosation of tyrosine, cysteine residues. NO, which a highly reactive radical, is spreadable and its life is very short. L-arginine is converted to citrulline by NO production and is a substrate for NOS. NOS2 is expressed in macrophages, neutrophils, endothelial cells, vascular smooth muscle cells and cardiomyocytes. The competitive inhibition of endogenous methylarginine regulates the substrate level in NOS isoforms. Oxidative stress plays an important role in AF pathogenesis. NOS enzymes can be decomposed and transferred from NO production to superoxide anion, strong free radicals and oxidation. Therefore, NOSs that are associated with oxidative stress are important in AF pathogenesis. In the case development of AF, left atrial endocardial NOS reduction occurs. Thus, a significant reduction in NO production occurs. Clinical cohorts were performed to investigate the relationship between AF development and eNOS gene polymorphisms. In a study with a Caucasian population that developed AF, it was determined that eNOS T-786C, G894T and 4a/4b gene polymorphisms did not have genetic risk factors in the development of AF. In another study, while CC genotype of eNOS T-786C polymorphism was found to be a genetic risk factor for homocysteine concentrations, there was no significant relationship between this polymorphism and the risk of developing AF. In another study conducted with heart failure and AF patients, 894TT genotype of G894T gene polymorphism was determined as a genetic risk factor in development of AF. In a study conducted by Giusti et al., eNOS T-786C gene polymorphism was found to be associated with a decrease in eNOS gene promoter activity. Furthermore, in the same study, this polymorphism was found to be an independent risk factor for plasma homocysteine concentrations [7–9]. It is presented primer sequences that used to determine eNOS T-786, G894T, Intron 4a/4b gene polymorphisms in **Table 3**.

4. Endothelin 2 A985G gene polymorphism

AF is an important complication of hypertrophic cardiomyopathy and is observed in approximately 20% of patients with hypertrophic cardiomyopathy. Hemodynamic changes following

Genes	Primer	Primer sequences
Endothelin 2 A985G gene	Forward	5'-ACAAACCAGGAGCAACCGTG-3'
	Reverse	5'-AGGGAATGAGGGTGCAAGAA-3'
	G allele-specific probe	5'-VIC-CCCTGGAGACTGGA-MGB-3'
	A allele-specific probe	5'-FAM-CCGGAGGCTGGAT-MGB-3'

PCR, polymerase chain reaction.

Table 4. Sequence of primers for endothelin 2 A985G gene polymorphism.

sympathetic or parasympathetic activation play an important role in AF triggering. In a study conducted by Thomson et al., hypertension was reported to induce triggering in developing of AF in patients with hypertrophic cardiomyopathy. Since myocardial hypertrophy is present in patients with hypertrophic cardiomyopathy, the left ventricular space is small in these patients. Thus, a decrease occurs in venous conversion and intravascular volume. As a result of this, in the patients with hypertrophic cardiomyopathy, low heart debit and various symptoms arise. Cheung et al. suggested that AF could be induced in the study they performed. Endothelin 2, which constricts the systemic vessels, protects venous return and prevents hypertension that may develop. Acute hypertension causes an increase in sympathetic nerve activity. Hypertension can occur in hypertrophic cardiomyopathy. A vasoconstrictor may show protective effect against AF in hypertrophic cardiomyopathy. Proximal AF is more common in hypertrophic cardiomyopathy than in other structural heart diseases. This monogenic disorder is a disorder affecting left ventricular hypertrophy in patients with hypertrophic cardiomyopathy. These disorders result from mutations in genes encoding the sarcomeric proteins. In a study conducted by Sharma et al., it has been shown that the endothelin 2 gene may be effective in the development of hypertension, and that this gene is expressed to in human atrial tissue. Endothelin 2 gene is localized on chromosome 1p34. It has been suggested that there is a significant relationship between hemodynamic changes and polymorphisms occurring in endothelin 2 gene in patients with essential hypertension. The functional role of endothelin 2 A985G gene polymorphism is not known precisely. mRNA stability is affected by variations in 3'-UTR. Thus, endothelin 2 transcription and translation may be affected in the endothelin 2 A985G gene polymorphism. Differences in A985 allele frequencies are observed in studies with different populations. Endothelin 2 A985G gene polymorphism plays a protective role for A985 allelic cardiovascular diseases, but this allele may trigger AF development in hypertrophic cardiomyopathic patients. In a study conducted by Nagai T et al., The endothelin 2 A985T allele has been shown to be a genetic risk factor for the development of AF in hypertrophic cardiomyopathic patients [10]. It is presented primer sequences that used to determine Endothelin 2 A985G gene polymorphism in **Table 4**.

5. Connexins gene polymorphisms

AF can also occur when there is or no structural heart disease. Most of the foci that cause AF are at the site where combine the cardiomyocytes and vascular smooth muscle cells are located near the pulmonary venules. Connexins (Cx) are gap junction proteins and play an important role in direct cell-cell interactions in the majority of the tissues of the body in electrical conduction in the heart. It is known that there are 20 different Cxs in humans, and each Cxs create channels with different

Genes	Primer	Primer sequences
Cx37 1019 C>T	Forward	5'-CTGGACCCACCCCCTCAGAATGGCCAAAGA-3'
	Reverse	5'-AGGAAGCCGTAGTGCCTGGTGG-3'
Cx40 G-44A	Forward	5'-CCCTCTTTTTAATCGTATCTGTGGC-3'
	Reverse	5'-GGTGGAGGGAAGAAGACTTTTAG-3'

PCR, polymerase chain reaction; Cx, connexin.

Table 5. Sequence of primers for the connexins.

characteristics and specific expression patterns. The polymorphisms occur in gap junction channels and in Cx proteins that play a role in action potential spread. Variants that occur in genes encoding variants that occur in genes encoding Cx40 and Cx37 that contribute to pulmonary vein-arrhythmogenic affect gene expression and function. Cx40 and Cx37 that contribute to pulmonary vein-arrhythmogenic affect gene expression and function. Variants that occur in genes encoding Cx40 and Cx37 that contribute to pulmonary vein-arrhythmia affect gene expression and function. The Cx40 gene is encoded by GJA5 and is expressed in endothelial cells, coronary vascular smooth muscle cells, atrial cardiomyocytes and cardiac conduction systems. In GJA5, the TATA box sequence also changes is the result of the single nucleotide polymorphism found in the promoter region. Cx40 gene modulates broad mRNA levels and is known to be associated with AF. In a previous study, Cx40-26G>A gene polymorphism-26G allele was identified as a genetic risk factor in patients with cardiomyopathy AF. In a study performed by Carballo et al., Cx40-26G>A gene polymorphism was found to affect protein expression levels in cardiomyocytes and this polymorphism was associated with structural AF. There are significant relationships between polymorphisms occurring in GJA5 in the Cx40 gene and susceptibility to AF. Somatic mutations in the Cx40 gene have also been associated with idiopathic AF. The Cx43 gene is also encoded by GJA1 and is expressed by ventricular, atrial cardiomyocytes, vascular smooth muscle cells, endothelial cells, monocytes and macrophages. Other genes and polymorphisms associated with polymorphisms in the CX43 gene have also been reported to be effective in the development of AF. The Cx37 gene is encoded by GJA4 and is found in endothelial cells, pulmonary and vascular smooth muscle cells, monocytes/macrophages and platelets. Polymorphisms occurring in GJA4 in the Cx37 gene are associated with atherosclerosis and coronary heart disease, and these polymorphisms have an effect on monocyte adhesion. Thus, they are important in the regulation of local inflammation. Systemic and local inflammation may play a role in the development of AF before or after surgery in some cases. The 1019 C>T gene polymorphism in the CX37 gene in GJA4 is characterized by proline/serine (P319S) substitution at position 319 in the cytoplasmic tail of the Cx37 gene. As a result, channel conductivity and permeability change. Cx37 1019 C>T gene polymorphism is also associated with platelet aggregation or monocyte adhesion. Due to the effect of this polymorphism on monocyte adhesion, sensitivity to non-structural AF may change [11–13]. It is presented primer sequences that used to determine Cx37 1019 C>T, Cx40 G-44A gene polymorphisms in **Table 5**.

6. Gamma-glutamyl carboxylase gene polymorphism

Warfarin, an oral anticoagulant, is used in the correction of various thromboembolitic disorders such as prosthetic heart valves, deep vein thrombosis and pulmonary embolism.

Genes	Forward primer (5′–3′)	Reverse primer (5′–3′)
rs699664	AGTGGCCTCGGAAGCTGGT	ACACAGGAAACACTGGGCTGAG
rs2592551	GGACTTAGAAAGGAACGGATGA	CTTGAGAAAAGGCAAAGCAGAC

PCR, polymerase chain reaction; SNP, single nucleotide polymorphism; GGCX, gamma-glutamyl carboxylase.

Table 6. Primer sequences used in PCR for GGCX.

Thromboembolism or bleeding may develop as a result of inadequate or excessive intake of warfarin. Discomforts such as stroke and systemic thromboembolism can be reduced with anticoagulant treatments. Factors such as age, body size, environment, interacting drugs and gene polymorphisms are effective at warfarin dose requirements. Stable warfarin dose is affected by gene polymorphisms such as single nucleotide gene polymorphism. These polymorphisms play a role in the modulation of warfarin pharmacodynamics and pharma-cokinetics. Gamma carbon carboxylation occurs on gamma glutamic acids. Gamma-glutamyl carboxylase (GGCX) found in the endoplasmic reticulum membrane oxidizes vitamin K-2,3 epoxite reduced vitamin K. Therefore, functional vitamin K-dependent clotting factors (II, VII, IX and X) are produced by this enzyme. GGCX catalyzes the biosynthesis of vitamin K-dependent clotting factors. Thus, this enzyme affects warfarin metabolism. Warfarin metabolism, one of the most frequently used anticoagulants in clinical therapy, is affected by the GGCX enzyme. GGCX is a gene that plays an important role in the individual differences of warfarin response. Warfarin is a common anticoagulant that a narrow therapeutic range. Genetic factors that play an important role in warfarin dose requirements include GGCX gene polymorphisms. GGCX gene that consisted of 15-exon is located on human chromo-some 2p12. It has been reported that there is a relationship between polymorphisms occurring in the GGCX gene and warfarin dose variability. GGCX rs11676382, rs12714145, rs10654848 and rs699664 gene polymorphisms are the most common polymorphisms of the GGCX gene. GGCX rs11676382 (C>G) gene polymorphism found in intron 14 was found to be associated with low Warfarin dose requirements in the Caucasus. In intron 2, GGCX rs12714145 (3261G>A) gene polymorphism was found to have more warfarin dose requirements in Chinese patients with the AA genotype. In Caucasians and African Americans, there is a significant relation-ship between GGCX rs10654848 microsatellite (DNA repeats) gene polymorphism in intron 6 and high warfarin dose requirements. GGCX rs699664 gene polymorphism, characterized by a G/A base substitution at the 8th exon. This displacement results in the arginine/glutamine amino acid exchange at position 325. In Japanese and Chinese patients, a significant relation-ship was determined between this polymorphism and high warfarin dose requirements. In contrast, in Caucasians or African Americans, this gene polymorphism was found not to be associated with warfarin dose. In AF patients, it was determined that GGCX rs699664 gene polymorphism was significantly correlated with GA, AA genotypes and high warfarin dose requirements. Another polymorphism associated with warfarin dose in patients with AF is the GGCX rs2592551 gene polymorphism. The effect of GGCX rs2592551 gene polymorphism on the warfarin dose was investigated in a study conducted by Kamali et al. in a population living in the Xinjiang region (region of multiple ethnic communities of Khan, Uyghur, Kazakh, Hui, Kyrgyz, Mongol and Tajik). In this study, CT and TT genotypes of GGCX rs2592551 gene polymorphism were found to be associated with higher warfarin dose requirements than CC genotype in patients with AF [14, 15]. It is presented primer sequences that used to determine GGCX rs699664, rs2592551 gene polymorphisms in **Table 6**.

7. G-protein β3 subunit C825T gene polymorphism

G-protein β3 subunit C825T gene polymorphism plays an important role in the change of electrophysiological properties of human atrium. This polymorphism occurs in 10th exon of gene, which encodes the G-protein β3 subunit. It has been determined by Siffert et al. that this polymorphism is a genetic risk factor in the development of hypertension. Increased human atrial internal rectifier regulatory potentials have been associated with the TT genotype of G-protein β3 subunit C825T gene polymorphism. There is also a significant relationship between the TT genotype of the G-protein β3 subunit C825T gene polymorphism and the increased internal rectifier flow and reduced acetylcholine stimulating potassium flux in the human atrium. In the European white population, 825 T allele of G-protein β3 subunit C825T gene polymorphism was found to be significantly associated with various cardiovascular disorders such as increased obesity, hypertension, left ventricular hypertrophy and coronary artery disease. In a study performed by Schreieck et al., heterozygote T and homozygote T allele carriage were found to be low risk factors for AF development. G-protein β3 subunit the TT and CT genotypes of the C825T gene polymorphism play an important role in atrial cellular electrophysiological changes. In a study conducted by Dobrev et al., it was determined that TT genotype of this polymorphism correlates with the downregulation of acetylcholine mRNA transcripts in human atrial myocytes. Although there is no relationship between G-protein β3 subunit C825T gene polymorphism and any arrhythmia, in some studies this polymorphism has been associated with the risk of developing AF. In conclusion, gene polymorphisms encoding ion channels are very important in AF pathogenesis. Identification of these polymorphisms will elucidate the multigenic mechanism of AF predisposition [16]. It is presented primer sequences that used to determine G-protein β3 subunit C825T gene polymorphism in **Table 7**.

Genes	Primer	Primer sequences
G-protein β3 subunit C825T gene	Forward	5'-TTCTCCCACGAGAGCATCATCT-3'
	Reverse	5'-GTCGTCGTAGCCAGCGAATAGTA-3'
	Allele 825C probe	5'-CATCACGTCCGTGGCCTTCTCC-3'
	Allele 825T probe	5'-CATCACGTCTGTGGCCTTCTCCCT-3'

PCR, polymerase chain reaction.

Table 7. Sequence of primers for G-protein β3 subunit C825T gene polymorphism.

8. Polymorphisms in the genes coding ion channels

8.1. KCNN3 rs13376333 gene polymorphism

Differences in populations due to myocardial membrane stability, conduction routes or genetic polymorphisms are important factors in predisposing to AF development. In recent association studies, gene polymorphisms found on chromosomes 4q25, 16q22 and 1q21 have been identified as genetic risk factors for AF development. Moreover, these genetic variants are more important in the development of early onset AF. The relationship between these gene polymorphisms and the risk of developing AF has been explored in different populations. From these populations, in one Chinese and European origin considerable differences have been found in terms of these polymorphisms. rs2200733 on the 4q25 chromosome and rs106261 gene polymorphisms on the 16q22 chromosome have been observed quite often in the Chinese population in particular. However, the relationship between the rs7193343 gene polymorphism on the 16q22 chromosome and the risk of developing AF was not significant in the Chinese Han population. In a study conducted by Ellinor et al. with the European population, KCNN3 single nucleotide gene polymorphism, which is associated with AF in the new genetic locus, has been discovered in the potassium medium/small conductance calcium-activating channel. The KCNN3 gene encodes voltage-independent calcium and activated potassium channels. The KCNN3 rs13376333 gene polymorphism is located between the first and second exons of the KCNN3 gene. There are three subtypes of potassium channels as SK1, SK2 and SK3. Atrial myocytes are formed by the subunits of these channels to form heteromultimeric complexes. The expression of SK3 channels is similar to the expressions of SK1 and SK2 channels. There are studies showing that the relationship between these SK channels and AF is significant. However, more studies are needed to determine the role of SK3 channels in AF development. Studies were also conducted in the Asian population to investigate AF associations with KCNN3 gene polymorphisms, which are the ionic channel gene identified in AF GWAS. However, a large number of replication studies are needed to determine this relationship. In a study conducted by Chang et al., KCNN3 rs13376333 gene polymorphism in the Taiwanese population was found to be an important risk factor for the development of AF. Also Ellinor et al. showed that there is a significant association between AF and KCNN3 rs13376333 gene polymorphism. In a study conducted with Chinese Han population, KCNN3 rs13376333 gene polymorphism has not been identified as a genetic risk factor in the development of AF. In Taiwan and China populations, the T allele of KCNN3 rs13376333 gene polymorphism was observed at a significantly lower frequency [17].

8.2. SCN10A gene polymorphism

Voltage-gated sodium channels play an important role in impulse generation and conduction during the rising phase of action potential in excitable cells. There are sodium channel isoforms in the heart. These channels include voltage-gated sodium 1.1, voltage-gated sodium 1.3, voltage-gated sodium 1.5 ($Na_v1.5$), voltage-gated sodium 1.6 and voltage-gated sodium 1.8 channels. The $Na_v1.5$ encoded by SCN5A is responsible for the regulation of cardiac conduction. The Nav1.5 channel plays a very important role in cardiac impulse spread. As a result of the activation of sodium channels, the cardiac action potential is rapidly increasing. Each sodium channel consists of an α subunit and modulating β subunits. The α subunit of the NaV1.5 channel is encoded by the SCN5A gene. Each of the Nav1.5 α subunit consists of 4 homologous domains (DI-DIV) with 6 transmembrane alpha helices (S1-S6). The S1-S4 domains are repeatable and these domains constitute the voltage sensing areas of the channel. The functional pore and selectivity filter of the sodium channel consists of S5, S6 and S5-S6 loops. More than 300 mutations have been identified in the SCN5A gene. SCN5A mutations determined to be associated with Brugada Syndrome (BrS) lead to variable reductions in the sodium flow inward with channel transit changes. These channel passing changes delayed activation, increased inactivation, slow recovery from inactivation, or impaired exchange of channel. As a result, decrease in expression occurs in the cell membrane. Consequently, these mechanisms cause loss of function in the cardiac sodium channel. The most common genotype found among BrS patients stems from mutations in the SCN5A gene. As a result of these mutations occurring in the gene, there is a loss of function in the cardiac sodium channel through different mechanisms. Depolarization or repolarization of cardiac action potential may be affected by due to reduced sodium current. Nevertheless, the underlying pathophysiological mechanism of the BrS phenotype is still being discussed [18]. BrS is defined as a disease characterized by sudden cardiac death characterized by a right bundle branch with an ST segment elevation in leads V1 and V2 in 1992. This syndrome was found to be associated with sudden cardiac death, especially in young men [19]. BrS, determined to be genetic, is a cardiac electrical disorder. BrS, an arrhythmogenic and autosomal dominant inherited cardiac syndrome, is characterized by typical electrocardiographic changes. In a study conducted in the Chinese population, localized in the domain II S4 segment of NaV1.5 α subunit protein, a new mutation, L812Q mutation, has been described. In this study, it was shown that this mutation improved the sodium channel inactivation process and disrupted the membrane expression of the canal in BrS patients [18]. In a Dutch population study, it was determined that SCN5A gene mutations, which cause loss of function in BrS patients, are associated with dilation and deterioration in contractile function of both ventricles [20]. In another study, SCN5A showed a high penetrance for BrS in a large family with the E1784K mutation. In addition, in the same study, overexpressing phenotypes of BrS were shown in E1784K and H558R carriers after the fourth decades of their lifes [21]. There is an effect in the cardiac electrophysiological properties of sodium-gated voltage channel 1.8 via the effect intrinsic on cardiac ganglion neurons. In the isolated ventricular myocardium, it is known that the sodium-gated voltage 1.8 channel is not expressed. In isolated intrinsic cardiac ganglia, there are immunoelectrochemical studies indicating that significant amounts of sodium-gated voltage 1.8 channels are expressed. Facer et al. have shown that sodium-gated voltage 1.8 channel immunoreactive sensory nerves are present in human atrial myocardium. Voltage-gated sodium 1.8 channel is encoded by SCN10A and is a tetradoxin (TTX)-resistant sodium channel. This channel is expressed in dorsal root ganglia, cranial sensory ganglion sensory neurons. The SCN10A gene, which contains 27 exons, is localized on chromosome 3q22.2. The SCN10A gene has been shown to be associated with cardiac transmission. Because the SCN10A gene plays a role in increasing the PR interval and QRS duration in the electrocardiogram. Therefore, it was found that there is a relation between SCN10A and AF development. The SCN10A sodium-gated voltage 1.8 channel plays an important role in modulating the induction of AF. Verkerk et al. have demonstrated that the SCN10A sodium-gated voltage 1.8 channel is present in intrinsic cardiac neurons. In a study conducted by Chambers et al., a significant relationship was found between SCN10A rs6795970 gene polymorphism and PR interval. SCN10A rs6795970 (G>A) gene polymorphism is a missense mutation and causes an A1073V amino acid substitution in the sodium-gated voltage channel 1.8 IDII/III intracellular cycle. In a study conducted by Ritchie et al., the G allele of SCN10A rs6795970 gene polymorphism was found to be a genetic risk factor for the development of AF. In another study performed by Sabbari et al., G allele of SCN10A rs6795970 gene polymorphism was associated with increased risk of AF. A significant association was found between the SCN10A rs6800541 gene polymorphism and AF development in the study conducted by Pfeufer et al. [22, 23].

8.3. KCNE1 G38S gene polymorphism

KCNE1 widely known as a potassium ion channel encoding gene for humans and it is localized on chromosome 21q22.1–21q22.2 encoding the subunit of the potassium ion channel (IKs).
KCNE1 plays an important role in atrial and ventricular repolarization. The KCNE1 gene was
discovered by Murai et al. in 1989. Studies have shown that KV7.1, the α subunit of the IKS current, plays an important role in AF pathogenesis. The regulatory β subunits of the IKS current
also bind to the KCNE1 gene. Biophysical properties of these β subunits of KV.71 can be altered
by expression together. The β subunits of IKS contain 130 amino acids, which is called the Mink
protein. Several single nucleotide gene polymorphisms have been identified in the KCNE1 gene.
The most common of these polymorphisms is the KCNE1 G38S (rs1805127 G>A, G38S) polymorphism. The KCNE1 gene polymorphism is characterized by a glycine or serine amino acid
substitution in the 38th position of the gene. As a result, stronger IKs flows occur. Various studies
have been carried out to demonstrate that the KCNE1 gene and polymorphisms are highly effective in AF pathogenesis. In a study conducted by Lai et al., a significant association was found
between the risk of developing AF in the Taiwanese population and the KCNE1 G38S gene polymorphism. Despite this conclusion in the Taiwanese population, it has been determined that
this polymorphism is not a genetic risk factor in the development of AF in the Chinese population. Studies conducted with European and Uighur populations have also found that KCNE1
G38S polymorphism is a risk factor associated with AF. A total of 14 studies were conducted to
investigate the relationship between KCNE1 G38S gene polymorphism and the risk of developing AF. In eight of these studies, a significant relationship was found between the risk of
developing KCNE1 G38S gene polymorphism and AF. However, no significant relationship was
determined in other six studies. In a meta-analysis study conducted by Jiang et al., to evaluate
the relationship between KCNE1 G38S polymorphism and AF, it is concluded the KCNE1 G38S
gene polymorphism increased AF risk. In a study carried out by Yadav et al., in the North Indian
population, KCNE1 G38S gene polymorphism was found to be not a risk factor for postoperative
AF development. In a study by Chen et al., it was found that the arrhythmia matrix is important

SNP rs	Forward primer (5′–3′)	Reverse primer (5′–3′)
KCNN3 rs13376333	TGAGAGCACCTGCAGACATC	GCAGCAAGAAGTGGGTCAAT
SCN10A-1 rs6795970	ATGACCCGAACTGACCTTCC	TGACGCTAAAATCCAGCCAGT
SCN10A-2 rs6795970	TGACAGAGGAGCAGAAGAAATACTACA	GTTGAGGCAGATGAGGACCA
KCNE1 rs1805127	GTGACGCCCTTTCTGACCAA	CCAGATGGTTTTCAACGACA
KCNE1 rs1892593	TGGGCTCTATTTTCAG	CCATTGGTCATTTTCC

PCR, polymerase chain reaction; SNP, single nucleotide polymorphism.

Table 8. Primer sequences used in PCR for polymorphisms in the genes coding ion channels.

at the onset or maintenance of AF. The arrhythmia matrix is formed by the interaction of proteins encoded by KCNE1 with other proteins. Therefore, the KCNE1 gene plays a very important role in regulating cardiac rhythm. Studies involving subgroup analyzes also found that the risk of developing AF in white populations with risk alleles was higher than in the Chinese population. The pathogenesis of AF is unknown. However, as a result of mutations in the genes encoding the ion channel, AF can develop due to a decrease in IKs. Environmental factors and genetic factors play a role in the pathogenesis of AF. It has been determined that different polymorphisms in genes encoding ion channels other than the KCNE1 G38S gene polymorphism may also be important risk factors for AF development [24, 25]. It is presented primer sequences that used to determine polymorphisms in the genes coding ion channels in **Table 8**.

9. RPL3L and MYZAP gene polymorphisms

A polygenic process involving transcription factors, cardiac ion channels, myocardial and cytoskeletal proteins plays an important role in AF pathogenesis. Based on the entire genome sequence, GWAS has shown that three low-frequency coding variants are effective in the development of AF. The myosin sarcomeric genes MYH6 and MYL4, the cytoskeletal gene PLEC, are these variants. MYH6, MYL4 and PLEC genes also encode cardiomyocyte structural components such as MYZAP. Ribosome activity can be specifically regulated in the cell via changes in the ribozyme protein composition. The eukaryotic ribosome consists of 4 different ribosomal RNAs and about 80 ribosomal proteins. This ribosome plays an important role in translating the messenger mRNA into a protein. Ribosomal proteins or genes encoding ribosome biogenesis factors may result in mutations leading to ribosomopathy, a hereditary disease. It is known that RPL3L-containing ribosomes may cause translational activity changes. Among RPL3L missense mutations, a negative regulator of muscle growth, p.Ala75Val and p.Gly12Arg mutations are important. Apart from these mutations, the RPL3L c.1167+1G>A mutation is involved in the impairment of the interaction of RPL3L with endoplasmic reticulum. As a result of these mutations, the risk of developing AF is increasing. Human Myozap mRNA is expressed primarily in the heart. Myozap regulates serum response factor signaling in the nucleus. This is why it plays an important role in cardiac signal transduction. Mutations in intercalated disk genes result in cardiomyopathies and sudden cardiac deaths that are a significant risk for AF. AF variants are defined in the genes coding for components of intercalated discs and in the vicinity of these genes. Seeger et al. found the MYZAP gene in the components of intercalated discs. Intercalated discs are a cell-cell contact structure that provides mechanical, electrical and chemical communication between cardiomyocytes. The risk of AF is also increasing as a result of MYZAP p.Gln254Pro gene polymorphism. In a previous study, there was a significant relationship between four low-frequency coding variants in the RPL3L and MYZAP genes and the risk of developing AF. The missense variant in MYZAP was identified as a genetic risk factor in the development of AF [26].

10. Gene polymorphisms and C-reactive protein levels related to inflammation

Several studies have been carried out to investigate the relationship between inflammation and AF. These studies have led to the conclusion that inflammation may cause AF or play an important role in the onset and maintenance of AF. Myocarditis, pericardiotomy and C-reactive protein (CRP) levels were associated with AF, a dysrhythmia, in studies conducted. However, in some other studies, it has been determined that there is a relationship between AF and the induction of inflammatory response. Previous studies have suggested that AF may be due to inflammatory processes and there is a significant relationship between the CRP levels and the risk of developing AF in these studies. A study performed by Lo et al. found a significant relationship between high basal CRP levels and increased postoperative AF risk. Non-Willebrand factor expression, which is effective in tissue factor, fibrinogen, factor VIII and prothrombic state, is induced by the IL-6 gene, which plays an important role in inflammation. Another study by Gaudino et al. found that −174 G/C polymorphism, a polymorphism in the promoter region of the interleukin-6 (IL-6) gene, was a significant effect on the inflammatory response and was associated with the risk of postoperative AF development. Also Marcus et al., in their study showed a significant relationship between increased IL-6 levels and the risk of developing AF. There is also a study showing that patients with high CRP levels have higher AF risk than patients with normal CRP levels [27].

11. Gene polymorphisms on chromosome 4q25

There are four unique nucleotide polymorphisms on the 4q25 chromosomal region, rs2200733, rs2220427, rs2634073 and rs10033464, and in studies conducted in European and Chinese populations, a significant relationship was found between these polymorphisms and the risk of developing AF. There are no known biological roles of these single nucleotide polymorphisms. These polymorphisms near to the homedomain transcription factor 2 (PITX2) gene and potentially alter the function of this factor. PITX2 is involved in the cardiac pathogenesis of ischemic and pulmonary venous access pathways. rs2200733 and rs13143308 that among the polymorphisms found on the 4q25 chromosome have also been identified as genetic risk factors for AF development. There are also several epidemiological cohorts recently showing a significant association between rs2200733, rs10033464 single nucleotide polymorphisms located in the 4q25 chromosome and AF development. In a recent study, rs2200733 polymorphism was found to be a genetic risk factor for AF development, proliferation and recurrence [28].

12. PRRX1 rs3903239 gene polymorphism

PRRX1 (paired-related HomeBox 1) is a gene encoding homedomain transcription factor that is expressed high in the developing heart. As a result of GWAS, the molecular mechanisms related to AF have been tried to be elucidated. In a recent meta-GWAS, significant correlations were found between the risk of developing rs3903239 polymorphism and AF on the 1q24 chromosome of the PRRX1 gene. In another study conducted with the Greek population, the role of the genetic interaction between PRRX1 rs3903239 and PITX2 rs2200733 gene polymorphisms in the development of AF was investigated and no significant interaction could be detected between these polymorphisms in AF patients. In addition, there was no significant difference in terms of PRRX1 rs3903239 allele frequencies and genotypes between AF patients and healthy controls in the same study. In another study conducted with the Chinese population, PRRX1 rs3903239 gene polymorphism was not detected as a significant genetic risk factor for AF [29].

13. β-fibrinogene 455G/A gene polymorphism

Various studies have been conducted to investigate the relationship between β-fibrinogen 455G/A polymorphism and ischemic stroke in different populations. In a study conducted by Kessler et al., the AA genotype of the β-fibrinogen 455G/A polymorphism was more observed in patients with major vascular infarction. In a study conducted by Nishiuma et al., in a Japanese population, A allele of β-fibrinogen 455G/A polymorphism was identified as an independent risk factor for hypertensive patients. In a study conducted by Martiskainen et al., a significant association was found between the A-allele and the lacunar infarction susceptibility in the β-fibrinogen 455G/A polymorphism. In a study conducted by Zhang et al., in the Chinese population, β-fibrinogen 455G/A polymorphism was found to be a genetic risk factor in the development of ischemic stroke. There are some meta-analysis studies showing that β-fibrinogen 455G/A polymorphism is associated with ischemic stroke in Chinese or Asian populations. A number of studies have been conducted to determine the association between this polymorphism and ischemic stroke, but no study has shown genetic effects in the pathogenesis of cardioembolic stroke in AF patients. The role of β-fibrinogen 455G/A polymorphism in cardioembolic stroke pathology is unclear. Promoter elements play an important role in regulating gene transcription. Transcription factor binding sites and transcription initiation rates can be varied by a promoter variant. β-fibrinogen 455G/A polymorphism has an important stimulatory effect on the rate of basal and induced transcription rate of the β-fibrinogen gene. There is a significant association between A allele of this polymorphism and increased promoter activity. β-Fibrinogen 455G/A polymorphism is one of the genetic polymorphisms associated with an increase in plasma fibrinogen. The increase in fibrinogen levels of individuals with A allele is greater than the increase in fibrinogen levels of individuals with G allele. Therefore, A allele of β-fibrinogen 455G/A polymorphism was found to be associated with higher fibrinogen level. Platelet aggregation, fibrinogen, an important determinant of blood viscosity, is a component that plays a role in the coagulation cascade. As a result of elevated fibrinogen levels, thrombosis progresses and coagulation increases. In animal studies, fibrinogen applications have been shown to increase thrombosis and embolic status at increasing doses. In addition, it is known that fibrinogen has been implicated in triggering various inflammatory processes. As a basic component of inflammation, fibrinogen can cause impairment of thrombus plaque and is effective in the development of ischemic stroke. As a result of all these events, hemorheological disorders occur. As a result of all these events, hemorheological disorders occur. Other polymorphisms that occur in the fibrinogen gene may also cause high fibrinogen concentrations such as β-fibrinogen 455G/A polymorphism β-fibrinogen 455G/A polymorphism has also been proven to be ineffective in the development of thrombotic events. In a study carried out by Xiaofeng Hu et al., in Chinese AF patients, proved that there is a relationship between increased risk of cardioembolic stroke and β-fibrinogen 455G/A polymorphism [30].

14. MTHFR (C677T and A1298C) and MTR A2756G gene polymorphisms

Hyperhomocysteinemia plays an important role in the pathogenesis of nonvalvular AF. Hyperhomocysteinemia develops as a result of polymorphisms occurring in genes encoding

Genes	Forward primer (5'–3')	Reverse primer (5'–3')
MTHFR C677T	biotinTGAAGGAGAAGGTGTCTGCGGGA	CCACTCCAGCATCACTCACT
MTHFR A1298C	biotinCAAGGAGGAGCTGCTGAAGA	CTTGAGAAAAGGCAAAGCAGAC
MTR A2756G	CATGGAAGAATATGAAGATATTAGAC	biotinGAACTAGAAGACAGAAATTCTCTA

PCR, polymerase chain reaction; SNP, single nucleotide polymorphism; MTHFR, methylenetetrahydrofolate reductase; MTR, methionine synthase reductase.

Table 9. Primer sequences used in PCR for MTHFR C677T and A1298C, MTR A2756G.

homocysteine metabolism. These polymorphisms are thought to be effective in the development of nonvalvular AF, which is the most common arrhythmia in clinical practice. Homocysteine is a highly reactive, sulfur-containing amino acid that occurs as a product of the essential amino acid methionine. Gene polymorphisms known to be associated with homocysteine occur in genes encoding enzymes that play a role in the metabolism of homocysteine. Of these polymorphisms, MTHFR C677T and A1298C gene polymorphisms are associated with a decrease in MTHFR enzyme activity. In addition to these polymorphisms, there is also the MTR A2756G gene polymorphism. Homocysteine plays an important role in the pathogenesis of AF and there are studies showing that there is a significant relationship between increased homocysteine levels and AF. In some studies, there was a significant relationship between MTHFR C677T gene polymorphism and increased plasma homocysteine levels in patients with low folate levels. There are few studies related to MTHFR A1298C and MTR A2756G polymorphisms. In a study conducted by Betti Guisti et al., there was a significant relationship between plasma total homocysteine levels and MTHFR C677T gene polymorphism genotype distributions in patients with nonvalvular AF. Furthermore, no significant relationship was observed between plasma total homocysteine levels and MTHFR 1298AA and MTR 2756GG genotypes in nonvalvular AF patients. Given the combined genotype distributions, it is known that the MTHFR C677T and A1298C gene polymorphisms are related to each other [31]. It is presented primer sequences that used to determine MTHFR (C677T and A1298C) and MTR A2756G gene polymorphisms in **Table 9**.

15. Conclusion

Different results have been obtained in gene polymorphism studies to explain the pathogenesis of AF in which environmental and genetic factors play a role together. Differences in the results of these studies may result from different selection criteria for patients and control groups. Moreover, the findings obtained from these studies are different from each other because they are carried out with different races and populations. Identification of genes associated with AF and polymorphisms that occur in these genes will allow us to have information about the underlying mechanisms of the disease in susceptibility to this disease. Identification of candidate genes that play a role in genetic susceptibility to AF will be mentor to the prevention of this disease and the development of new therapies for disease. In order to be able to explain the pathogenesis of AF and to develop appropriate therapies for this disease, comprehensive studies should be conducted with different populations and with a large number of patients and control groups.

Acknowledgements

This chapter was performed by Nevra Alkanli, Arzu Ay and Suleyman Serdar Alkanli in department of Biophysics of T.C. Halic University Medical Faculty, Trakya University Medical Faculty and Istanbul University Medical Faculty.

Conflict of interest

We declare that there is no conflict of interest with any financial organization regarding the material discussed in the chapter.

Author details

Nevra Alkanli[1]*, Arzu Ay[2] and Suleyman Serdar Alkanli[3]

*Address all correspondence to: nevraalkanli@halic.edu.tr

1 Department of Biophysics, Faculty of Medicine, T.C. Halic University, Istanbul, Turkey

2 Department of Biophysics, Faculty of Medicine, Trakya University, Edirne, Turkey

3 Department of Biophysics, Faculty of Medicine, Istanbul University, Istanbul, Turkey

References

[1] Jiang MH, Su YM, Tang JZ. Angiotensin-converting enzyme gene 2350 G/A polymorphism and susceptibility to atrial fibrillation in Han Chinese patients with essential hypertension. Clinics. 2013;**68**(11):1428-1432. DOI: 10.6061/clinics/2013(11)08

[2] Zhang XL, Wu LQ, Liu X. Association of angiotensin-converting enzyme gene I/D and CYP11B2 gene −344T/C polymorphisms with lone atrial fibrillation and its recurrence after catheter ablation. Experimental and Therapeutic Medicine. 2012;**4**:741-747. DOI: 10.3892/etm.2012.650

[3] Olesen MS, Nielsen MW, Haunsø S. Atrial fibrillation: The role of common and rare genetic variants. European Journal of Human Genetics. 2014;**22**:297-306. DOI: 10.1038/ejhg.2013.139

[4] Tsai CT, Lai LP, Lin JL. Renin-angiotensin system gene polymorphisms and atrial fibrillation. Circulation. 2004;**109**:1640-1646. DOI: 10.1161/01.CIR.0000124487.36586.26

[5] Shuxın H, Yingmin L, Damin H. Correlation of atrial fibrillation with renin-angiotensin-aldosterone system gene polymorphism. Acta Medica Mediterranea. 2017;**33**:275. DOI: 10.19193/0393-6384_2017_2_041

[6] Feng W, Sun L, Qu XF. Association of AGTR1 and ACE2 gene polymorphisms with structural atrial fibrillation in a Chinese Han population. Die Pharmazie. 2017;**72**:17-21. DOI: 10.1691/ph.2017.6752

[7] Bonilla IM, Sridhar A, Györke S. Nitric oxide synthases and atrial fibrillation. Frontiers in Physiology Cardiac Electrophysiology. 2012;**3**:3-105. DOI: 10.3389/fphys.2012.00105

[8] Moguib O, Raslan HM, Rasheed IA. Endothelial nitric oxide synthase gene (T786C and G894T) polymorphisms in Egyptian patients with type 2 diabetes. Journal of Genetic Engineering and Biotechnology. 2017;**15**:431-436. DOI: 10.1016/j.jgeb.2017.05.001

[9] Sivria N, Unlu A, Palabiyik O. Endothelial nitric oxide synthase intron 4a/b polymorphism in coronary artery disease in Thrace region of Turkey. Biotechnology & Biotechnological Equipment. 2014;**28**(6):1115-1120. DOI: 10.1080/13102818.2014.980030

[10] Nagai T, Ogimoto A, Okayama H. A985G polymorphism of the endothelin-2 gene and atrial fibrillation in patients with hypertrophic cardiomyopathy. Circulation Journal. 2007;**71**:1932-1936

[11] Carballo S, Pfenniger A, Carballo D. Differential association of Cx37 and Cx40 genetic variants in atrial fibrillation with and without underlying structural heart disease. International Journal of Molecular Sciences. 2018;**19**:295. DOI: 10.3390/ijms19010295

[12] Piťha J, Hubáček JA, Piťhová P. The connexin 37 (1019C>T) gene polymorphism is associated with subclinical atherosclerosis in women with type 1 and 2 diabetes and in women with central obesity. Physiological Research. 2010;**59**:1029-1032

[13] Shuxin H, Yingmin L, Huang D. Association of atrial fibrillation with gene polymorphisms of connexin 40 and angiotensin II receptor type 1 in Chongming adults of shanghai. International Journal of Clinical and Experimental Medicine. 2015;**8**(7):11803-11810

[14] Jiang NX, Xu YH, Xia JW. Impact of GGCX polymorphisms on warfarin dose requirements in atrial fibrillation patients. Turkish Journal of Medical Sciences. 2017;**47**:1239-1246. DOI: 10.3906/sag-1609-26

[15] Kamali X, Wulasihan M, Yang YC. Association of GGCX gene polymorphism with warfarin dose in atrial fibrillation population in Xinjiang. Lipids in Health and Disease. 2013;**12**:149

[16] Schreieck J, Dostal S, von Beckerath N. C825T polymorphism of the G-protein 3 subunit gene and atrial fibrillation: Association of the TT genotype with a reduced risk for atrial fibrillation. American Heart Journal. 2004;**148**:545-550. DOI: 10.1016/j.ahj.2004.03.024

[17] Chang SH, Chang SN, Hwang JJ. Significant association of rs13376333 in KCNN3 on chromosome 1q21 with atrial fibrillation in a Taiwanese population. Circulation Journal. 2012;**76**:184-188. DOI: 10.1253/circj.CJ-11-0525

[18] Wang L, Meng X, Yuchi Z. De novo mutation in the SCN5A gene associated with Brugada syndrome. Cellular Physiology and Biochemistry. 2015;**36**:2250-2262. DOI: 10.1159/000430189

[19] Juang JMJ, Horie M. Genetics of Brugada syndrome. Journal of Arrhythmia. 2016; **32**:418-425

[20] van Hoorn F, Campian ME, Spijkerboer A. SCN5A mutations in Brugada syndrome are associated with increased cardiac dimensions and reduced contractility. PLoS One. 2012;**7**(8):e42037. DOI: 10.1371/journal.pone.0042037

[21] Veltmann C, Hector B-M, Wolpert C. Further insights in the most common SCN5A mutation causing overlapping phenotype of long QT syndrome, Brugada syndrome, and conduction defect. American Heart Association. 2016;**5**:e003379. DOI: 10.1161/ JAHA.116.003379

[22] Wu H, Juan X, Chen S. Association of SCN10A polymorphisms with the recurrence of atrial fibrillation after catheter ablation in a Chinese Han population. Scientific Reports. 2017;**7**:44003. DOI: 10.1038/srep44003

[23] Roman AC, Pinto FM, Subirán N. The voltage-gated sodium channel Nav1.8 is expressed in human sperm. PLoS One. 2013;**8**(9):e76084. DOI:10.1371/journal.pone.0076084

[24] Yadav S, Akhtar S, Agarwal SK. Genetic association of KCNE1G38S polymorphism in postoperative atrial fibrillation of North Indian population: A case-control study. Biomedical and Pharmacology Journal. 2017;**10**(3):1055-1060. DOI: 10.13005/bpj/1202

[25] Yao J, Ma YT, Xie X. Association of KCNE1 genetic polymorphisms with atrial fibrillation in a Chinese Han population. Genetic Testing and Molecular Biomarkers. 2012;**16**(11):1343-1346. DOI: 10.1089/gtmb.2012.0149

[26] Thorolfsdottir RB, Sveinbjornsson G, Sulem P. Mutations in RPL3L and MYZAP increase risk of atrial fibrillation. bioRxiv. [preprint first posted online]. 2017;**21**. DOI: 10.1101/223578

[27] Galea R, Cardillo MT, Caroli A. Inflammation and C-reactive protein in atrial fibrillation cause or effect? Texas Heart Institute Journal. 2014;**41**(5):461-468. DOI: 10.14503/ THIJ-13-3466

[28] Virani SS, Brautbar A, Lee VV. Usefulness of single nucleotide polymorphism in chromosome 4q25 to predict in-hospital and long-term development of atrial fibrillation and survival in patients undergoing coronary artery bypass grafting. The American Journal of Cardiology. 2011;**107**:1504-1509. DOI: 10.1016/j.amjcard.2011.01.026

[29] Letter to the Editor. PRRX1 Rs3903239 polymorphism and atrial fibrillation in a Greek population. Hellenic Journal of Cardiology. 2018:1-2. [Epub ahead of print]. DOI: 10.1016/j. hjc.2018.01.005

[30] Hu X, Wang J, Li Y. The β-fbrinogen gene 455G/A polymorphism associated with cardioembolic stroke in atrial fbrillation with low CHA2DS2-VaSc score. Scientific Reports. 2017;**7**:17517. DOI: 10.1038/s41598-017-17537-1

[31] Giusti B, Gori AM, Marcucci R. Role of C677T and A1298C MTHFR, A2756G MTR and −786 C/T eNOS gene polymorphisms in atrial fibrillation susceptibility. PLoS ONE. 2007;**2**(6): e495. DOI: 10.1371/journal.pone.0000495

8

Idiopathic Ventricular Arrhythmias

Takumi Yamada

Abstract

Idiopathic ventricular arrhythmias (VAs) occur with a mechanism that is unrelated to myocardial scar. Idiopathic VAs most commonly occur in patients without structural heart disease, but can occur in those with structural heart disease. Idiopathic VAs present as a sustained or a non-sustained ventricular tachycardia or premature ventricular contractions. Imaging examinations such as echocardiography, nuclear tests, and cardiac magnetic resonance imaging are helpful for excluding any association of an idiopathic VA occurrence with myocardial scar. For the past two decades, the sites of idiopathic VA origins, commonly endocardial but sometimes epicardial, have been increasingly recognized. Idiopathic VAs usually originate from specific anatomical structures and exhibit characteristic electrocardiograms based on their anatomical background. Idiopathic VAs are basically benign, but they require medical treatment or catheter ablation when idiopathic VAs are symptomatic, frequent, or cause tachycardia-induced cardiomyopathy. This book chapter describes the up-to-date information on the prevalence of idiopathic VA origins relevant to the anatomy, diagnosis, and treatment of idiopathic VAs.

Keywords: idiopathic, ventricular tachycardia, anatomy, diagnosis, treatment

1. Introduction

Idiopathic ventricular arrhythmias (IVAs) present as ventricular tachycardias (VTs) or premature ventricular contractions (PVCs) whose mechanisms are not associated with a myocardial scar. IVAs commonly occur in patients without structural heart disease (SHD), but can occur in those with SHD [1–3]. Classically, VTs originating from the right ventricular outflow tract (RVOT) and the left posterior fascicle are well known as IVAs. However, for the past two decades, IVAs originating from other endocardial and also epicardial sites have been increasingly recognized (**Figure 1**) [3]. IVAs usually originate from the specific anatomical

	RV	**LV**	
Outflow tract region			
Supravalvular	PA	Aorta	
Endocardial	RVOT	LVOT (AMC)	**LV ostium**
Epicardial		LV summit (GCV, AIVV)	
Annuli	TA (Peri-Hisian)	MA	
Fascicles		LPF >> LAF Upper septum	
Intracavital	PAM Moderator band	PPAM >> APAM	
Muscle bands	Infundibular muscles (Parietal band + Septal band)		
Epicardium		Crux (MCV)	

Figure 1. Idiopathic ventricular arrhythmia origins. AIVV, anterior interventricular vein; AMC, aorto-mitral continuity; APAM, anterolateral papillary muscle; GCV, great cardiac vein; LAF, left anterior fascicle; LPF, left posterior fascicle; LV, left ventricle; LVOT, LV outflow tract; MA, mitral annulus; MCV, mid-cardiac vein; PA, pulmonary artery; PAM, papillary muscle; PPAM, posteromedial papillary muscle; RV, right ventricle; RVOT, RV outflow tract; TA, tricuspid annulus.

structures and exhibit characteristic electrocardiograms based on their anatomical background. Basically, IVAs are benign and not life-threatening, but are often symptomatic and also can cause tachycardia-induced cardiomyopathy [4, 5]. Therefore, it is important for cardiologists to update their knowledge about IVAs. This chapter describes the current expertise on the prevalence of IVA origins relevant to the anatomy, diagnosis, and treatment of IVAs.

2. Prevalence of IVA origins relevant to the anatomy

The sites of IVA origins have been identified by electrophysiological mapping and confirmed by successful catheter ablation. The most common site of IVA origins is the ventricular outflow tract [1, 6]. IVAs originate more often from the RVOT than from the left ventricular outflow tract (LVOT). In the RVOT, the septum is a more common site of IVA origins than the free wall. The most common site of IVA origins in the LVOT is the aortic root followed by the sites underneath the aortic sinus cusps (ASCs) (**Figure 2**) [7, 8]. Especially, the site underneath the left coronary cusp (LCC) is located in front of the mitral annulus (MA) and is termed the aorto-mitral continuity (AMC). The MA is also one of the major sites of IVA origins [9, 10]. The anteromedial aspect of the MA may overlap with the AMC. Anatomically, the aortic and mitral valves are in a direct apposition and attach to the elliptical opening at the base of the left ventricle (LV)

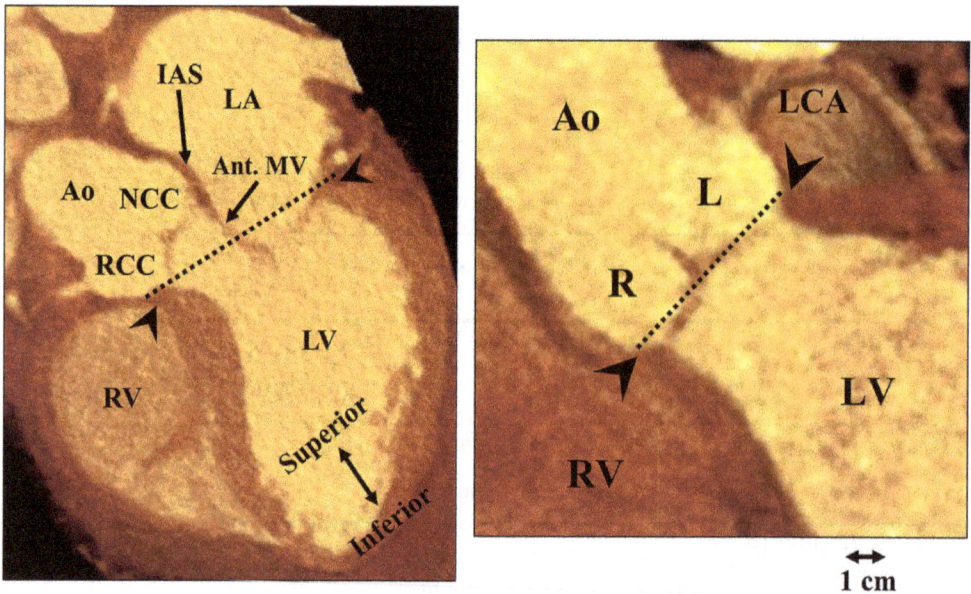

Figure 2. Two-dimensional computed tomography (CT) images showing the relationships between the ventricular myocardium and aortic sinus cusps. The arrowheads and dotted line in the left panel indicate the ostium of the left ventricle. The arrowheads in the right panel indicate the superior edge of the ventricular myocardium connecting with the left coronary cusp and right coronary cusp (RCC), and the dotted line the ventriculo-arterial junction. Ant, anterior; Ao, aorta; IAS, interatrial septum; L, left coronary cusp; LA, left atrium; LCA, left coronary artery; LV, left ventricle; MV, mitral valve; NCC, noncoronary cusp; R, right coronary cusp; RV, right ventricle. This figure was cited from Ref. [7] with permission.

known as the LV ostium [11, 12] (**Figure 2**). Because there is no myocardium between the aortic and the mitral valves (fibrous trigone), most idiopathic LV ventricular arrhythmias (VAs) can originate from along the LV ostium. The LV myocardium comes in direct contact with the aorta at the base of the ASCs (**Figure 2**). When IVAs arise from the most superior portion of the LV ostium (the aortic sinus of valsalva), they can be ablated within the base of the ASCs. It has been reported that some IVAs can be ablated from the junction (commissure) between the left and the right coronary cusps (L-RCC) [13]. In these VAs, catheter ablation from underneath the ASCs is often required for their elimination. Anatomically, the superior end of the LV myocardium makes a semicircular attachment to the aortic root at the bottom of the right and left coronary cusps. However, because of the semilunar nature of the attachments of the aortic valvular cusps, the superior end of the LV myocardium is located underneath the aortic valves at the L-RCC (**Figure 2**). Therefore, IVAs that can be ablated at the L-RCC should be classified into the same group as the VAs that can be ablated within the ASCs. In this setting, these IVAs may be defined as IVAs arising from the aortic root [7]. It has been reported that IVAs can rarely be ablated from within the noncoronary cusp of the aorta (NCC) [7, 14, 15]. Spatially, the aortic root occupies a central location within the heart, with the NCC anterior and superior to the paraseptal region of the left and right atria close to the superior atrioventricular junctions (**Figure 3**) [12]. In normal human hearts, the NCC is adjacent to the atrial myocardium on the epicardial aspect of the interatrial septum. When atrial tachycardias arise from that region of the atria, those atrial tachycardias can be ablated from within the NCC. It is considered that the NCC does not directly come in contact with the ventricular myocardium

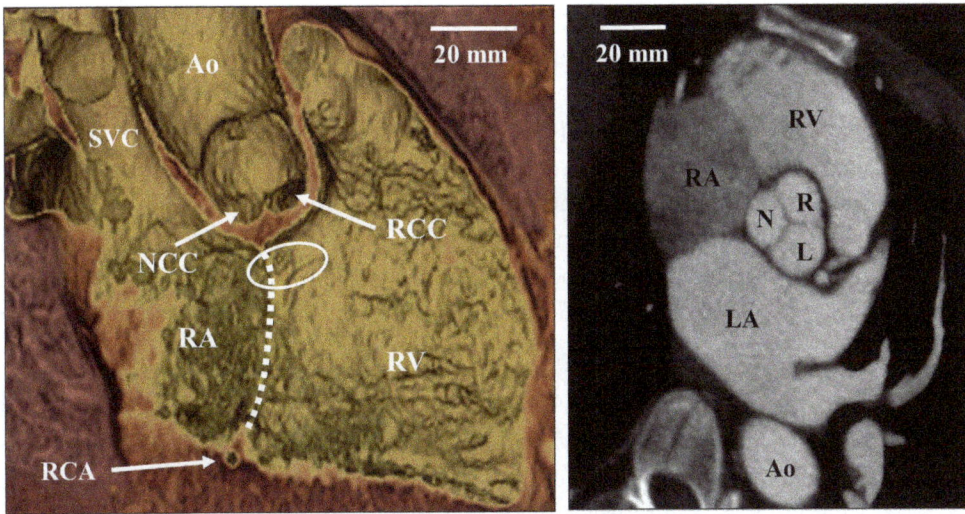

Figure 3. Two-dimensional (right panel) and three-dimensional (left panel) CT images. The dotted line indicates the tricuspid annulus and solid circle the right ventricular His bundle (HB) region. L, left coronary cusp; N, noncoronary cusp; RA, right atrium; RCA, right coronary artery; SVC, superior vena cava. The other abbreviations are as in the previous figures. This figure was cited from Ref. [15] with permission.

(**Figure 3**). However, it has been reported that some IVAs can be ablated from within the NCC [14]. The clinical observation that a noncoronary sinus of valsalva aneurysm can rupture into the right ventricle (RV), as well as the right atrium, supports the assumption that the NCC may be attached to the ventricular myocardium where IVAs can arise from. Some IVAs can be ablated from within the pulmonary sinus cusps [16]. The ventricular muscle is attached to the pulmonary sinus cusps (PSCs) in the RVOT like the ASCs in the LVOT. The ventricular muscle extends above the PSCs, but it should be noted that ventricular myocardial extensions never occurs in the aorta [12]. The ventricular muscle may appear to extend above the right coronary cusp (RCC) because of the specific nature of the interventricular septum. However, the superior end of the *left* ventricular muscle attaches to the RCC, and the *right* ventricular muscle attaching to the *left* ventricular muscle underneath the RCC runs in the interventricular septum up to the PSCs, which is located above the ASCs. In fact, the *right* ventricular muscle in the interventricular septum is separated from the RCC and aorta by a loose connective tissue. When IVAs arise from the ventricular muscle underneath the ASCs and PSCs or above the PSCs, catheter ablation within the ASCs and PSCs is required to cure those VAs because those VA origins are likely to be epicardial.

IVAs can originate from the atrioventricular annuli including the MA [9, 10] and tricuspid annulus (TA) [17]. IVAs originating from the MA and TA account for 5 and 8% of all IVAs, respectively. MA VAs can originate from any of the regions along the MA except the septal aspect where the fibrous trigone is located with no ventricular myocardium, but the antero-lateral and posteroseptal aspects of the MA are the most common and second most common sites of MA VA origins, respectively [9, 10]. TA VAs can originate from any regions along the TA, but more often originate from the septal aspect, especially in the anteroseptal or para-Hisian region than the free wall [17].

IVAs can arise from the intracavital structures including the papillary muscles (PAMs) [18–22] and moderator band (MB) [23]. PAM VAs account for approximately 7% of patients with IVAs [18–22]. LV PAM VAs are known to arise more commonly from the posteromedial PAM than from the anterolateral PAM [20]. The sites of the PAM VA origins are limited to the base of the PAMs. IVAs can rarely originate from the PMs in the RV [22]. IVAs can arise from all three RV PAMs, but half of them arise from the septal PAM [22]. It has been recently reported that the MB rarely can be a source of IVAs including PVCs, VTs, and ventricular fibrillation [23]. Anatomically, the MB is considered to be a part of the septomarginal trabeculation, crossing from the septum to the RV free wall and supporting the anterior PAM of the tricuspid valve (**Figure 4**) [23].

Most recently, it has been reported that IVAs can arise from the muscular bands in the RV [24, 25]. The RVOT is the most common site of IVA origins. In the RV, the TA is the second most common site of IVAs, and less commonly idiopathic VAs can originate from some RV muscles [3, 17, 22, 23]. Anatomically, the muscles of the RV may be divided into three groups: (1) trabeculae, (2) papillary muscles of the tricuspid valve, and (3) infundibular muscles (**Figure 5**). The muscles of the infundibulum are thick muscular bands, consisting of the septal and parietal bands. The junction of these two bands is often indicated by a raphe or a ridge extending from the superior papillary muscle to the nadir of the posterior pulmonary leaflet. This junction has been

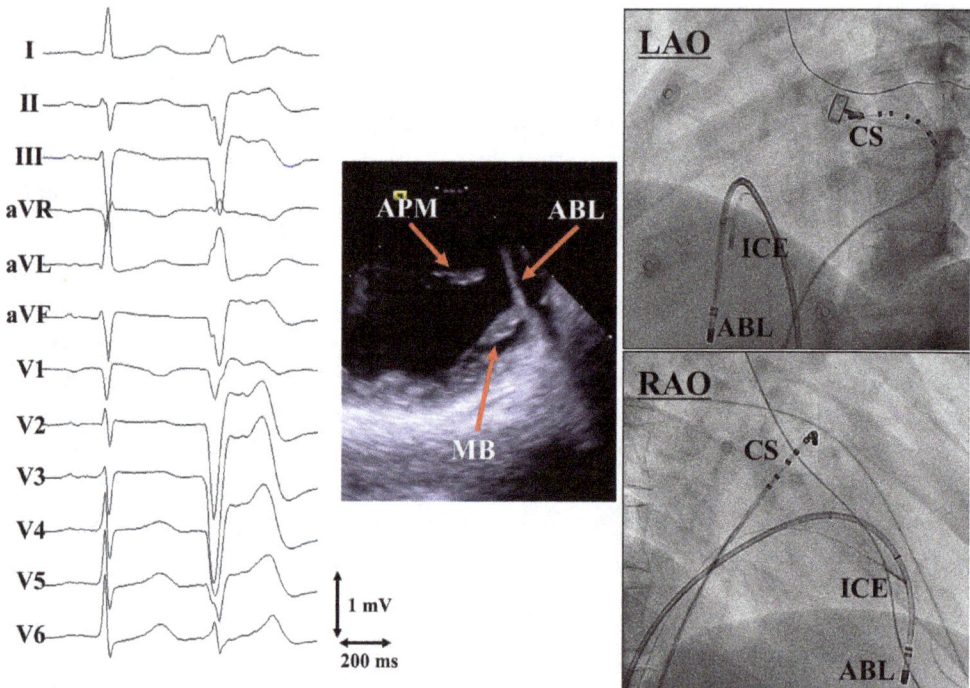

Figure 4. Twelve-lead electrocardiograms exhibiting a premature ventricular contraction originating from the moderator band (MB) (left panel) and an intracardiac echocardiographic image (middle panel) and fluoroscopic images (right panels) exhibiting the successful ablation site of the premature ventricular contraction originating from the MB. ABL, ablation catheter; APM, anterolateral papillary muscle; CS, coronary sinus; ICE, intracardiac echocardiography catheter; LAO, left anterior oblique; RAO, right anterior oblique. The other abbreviations are as in the previous figures. This figure was modified from Ref. [10] with permission.

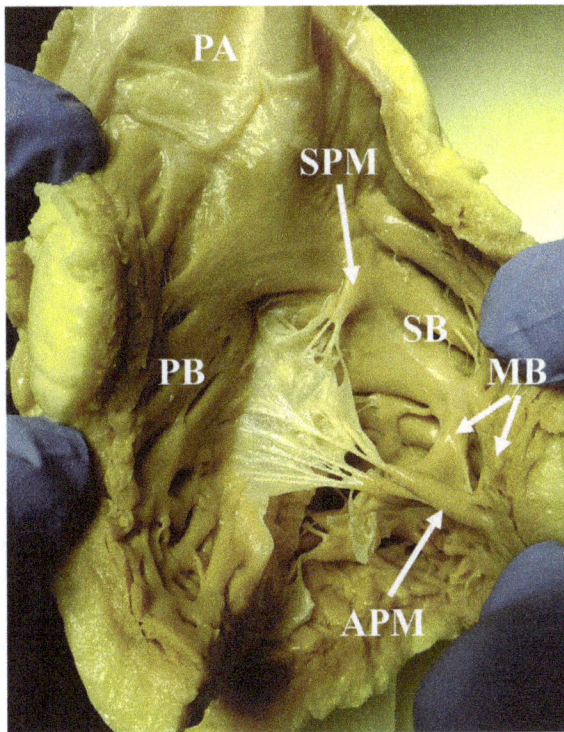

Figure 5. Autopsy heart exhibiting the infundibular muscles. PA, pulmonary artery; PB, parietal band; SB, septal band; SPM, superior papillary muscle. The other abbreviations are as in the previous figures. This figure was adapted from Ref. [25] with permission.

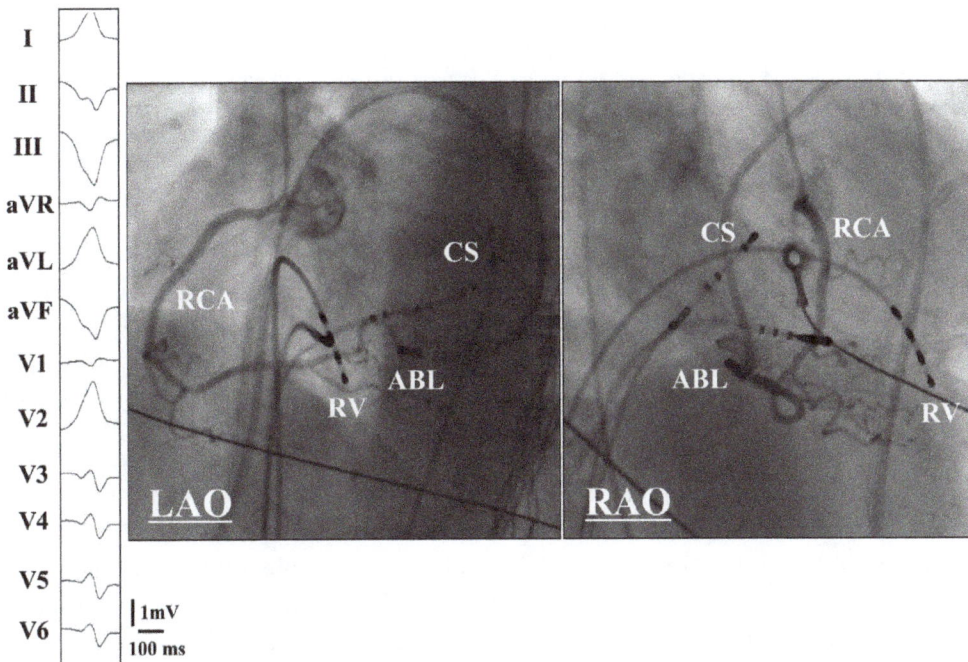

Figure 6. Twelve-lead electrocardiograms exhibiting the ventricular arrhythmia originating from the crux of the heart (left panel) and fluoroscopic images exhibiting its successful ablation site. The abbreviations are as in the previous figures. This figure was adapted from Ref. [30] with permission.

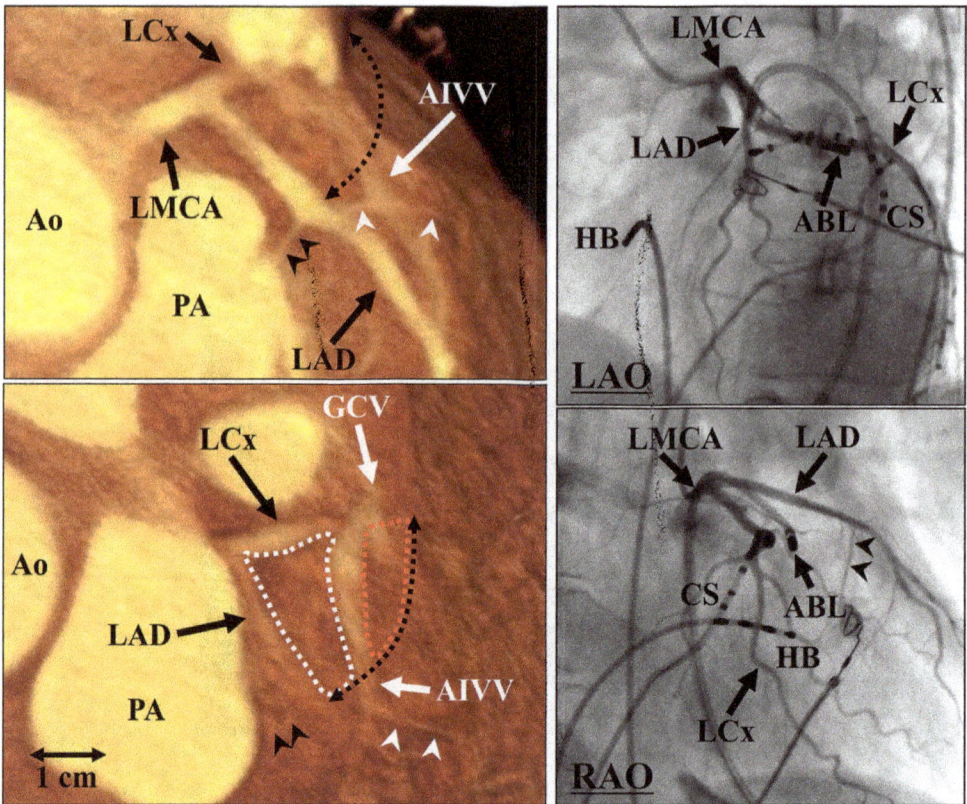

Figure 7. CT (left panels) and fluoroscopic (right panels) images exhibiting the LV summit. The LV summit was defined based on the fluoroscopy and coronary angiography as the region on the epicardial surface of the LV near the bifurcation of the left main coronary artery that is bounded by an arc (black dotted line) from the left anterior descending coronary artery (LAD) superior to the first septal perforating branch (black arrowheads) and anteriorly to the left circumflex coronary artery (LCx) laterally. The great cardiac vein (GCV) bisects the LV summit into a superior portion surrounded by the white dotted line (the *inaccessible area*) and an inferior portion surrounded by a red dotted line (the *accessible area*). The white arrowheads indicate the first diagonal branch of the LAD. AIVV, anterior interventricular cardiac vein; HB, His bundle; LMCA, left main coronary artery; PA, pulmonary artery. The other abbreviations are as in the previous figures. This figure was cited from Ref. [31] with permission.

termed the crista supraventricularis. An extension of the septal band is the MB, which usually extends inferiorly to the site of attachment of the anterior papillary muscle in the anterior wall. The parietal band extends across the tricuspid orifice onto the anterior wall, fading out above the area of the attachment of the anterior papillary muscle. IVAs rarely arise from the infundibular muscles, and parietal band IVAs are approximately three times as prevalent as septal band IVAs.

IVAs can arise from the Purkinje network, most commonly from the left posterior fascicle followed by the anterior and septal fascicles [21, 26, 27]. These IVAs most often present as reentrant VTs, but sometimes as VTs or PVCs with a focal mechanism. The left anterior fascicle runs along the MA. The left septal fascicle is located between the left anterior and posterior fascicles, and there is a normal variation in its origin and distribution. The peripheral Purkinje network extends to the surface of the PAMs and MB. Therefore, these VAs have to be differentiated from IVAs originating from the PAMs, MB, and atrioventricular annuli.

IVAs arise commonly from the endocardial side, but can arise from the epicardial side [27] and rarely from the intramural site [28, 29]. There are two major sites of origin of idiopathic epicardial VAs such as the crux of the heart [30] and LV summit [31]. Anatomically, the crux of the heart is formed by the junction of the atrioventricular groove and the posterior inter-ventricular groove and corresponds roughly to the junction of the middle cardiac vein and coronary sinus, near the origin of the posterior descending coronary artery (**Figure 6**) [30]. A region of the LV epicardial surface that occupies the most superior portion of the LV has been termed the LV summit by McAlpine (**Figure 7**) [11, 31]. The LV summit is bounded by the left anterior descending coronary artery and the left circumflex coronary artery. This region near where the great cardiac vein (GCV) ends and the anterior interventricular cardiac vein begins is one of the major sources of epicardial IVAs. The LV summit is bisected by the GCV into an area lateral to this structure that is accessible to epicardial catheter ablation (the *accessible area*) and a superior region that is inaccessible to catheter ablation due to the close proximity of the coronary arteries and a thick layer of epicardial fat that overlies the proximal portion of these vessels (the *inaccessible area*) [31]. The prevalence of LV summit VAs has been reported to account for 12% of idiopathic LV VAs. Among these VA origins, 70, 15, and 15% of them have been identified within the GCV, accessible area, and inaccessible area, respectively.

3. Diagnosis of IVAs

3.1. Imaging

IVAs are defined as VAs originating from normal ventricular myocardium. Therefore, any association of myocardial scar with an occurrence of VAs has to be excluded for a diagnosis of IVAs. Echocardiography and exercise stress testing are basic examinations to demonstrate no evidence of SHD. However, IVAs can occur in patients with SHD. If VAs originate away from the myocardial scar, they are considered idiopathic. Therefore, an imaging study such as echocardiography, nuclear test, or cardiac magnetic resonance imaging (cMRI) should be performed to locate the site of the scar in patients with SHD. Frequent IVAs can cause tachy-cardia-induced cardiomyopathy. When evidence of myocardial scar is excluded by a nuclear test or cMRI despite a reduced LV function, tachycardia-induced cardiomyopathy is likely to be present. A definite diagnosis of tachycardia-induced cardiomyopathy can be made when the LV function recovers after the IVAs are well treated by medication or catheter ablation.

3.2. Electrocardiogram

IVAs usually originate from specific anatomical structures and exhibit characteristic elec-trocardiograms (ECGs) based on their anatomical background. In general, the first clue in 12-lead surface electrocardiograms for predicting a site of an IVA origin is a bundle branch block pattern in lead V1. A right bundle branch block (RBBB) pattern clearly suggests an origin in the LV, whereas a left bundle branch block (LBBB) pattern suggests an origin in the RV or the interventricular septum. Second, an inferior axis (dominant R waves in leads II, III, and aVF) suggests an origin in the superior aspect of the ventricle, whereas a superior axis suggests an origin in the inferior aspect. A negative QRS polarity in lead I suggests an origin in the LV free wall [2, 9], and a QS pattern in lead V6 suggests an origin near the apex

(**Figures 4**, **8**, and **9**) [2, 21]. An R/S wave amplitude ratio of >1 in lead V6 suggests an origin in the base (ventricular outflow tract or annuli), whereas an R/S wave amplitude ratio of <1 suggests an origin in the middle of the ventricle (papillary muscles or left fascicles) (**Figures 4**, **8**, and **9**) [2, 21]. Twelve-lead ECGs are very helpful for predicting the likely epicardial VT origins (**Figures 10** and **11**). Because in human hearts, the Purkinje network that can quickly facilitate ventricular activation throughout the ventricles is located only in the subendocardium, ventricular activation from the epicardial origin requires more time to reach the Purkinje network, resulting in a slow onset of the QRS during epicardial VTs. Based on this mechanism, several parameters predicting epicardial VT origins have been proposed: a "pseudo-delta" wave duration of >34 ms, a QRS duration of >200 ms, a delayed intrinsicoid deflection of >85 ms, an RS complex duration of >121 ms, and a maximum deflection index (MDI) (calculated by dividing the shortest time from the QRS onset to the maximum deflection in any of the precordial leads by the total QRS duration) of >0.54 (**Figure 10**) [33, 34]. When ventricular activation propagates from an epicardial origin at the LV free wall or ventricular posterior wall, the total activation vector should go from a lateral toward medial or from an inferior toward superior direction, resulting in a QS pattern in lead I or lead aVF (**Figure 11**) [32]. On the other hand, when ventricular activation propagates from an

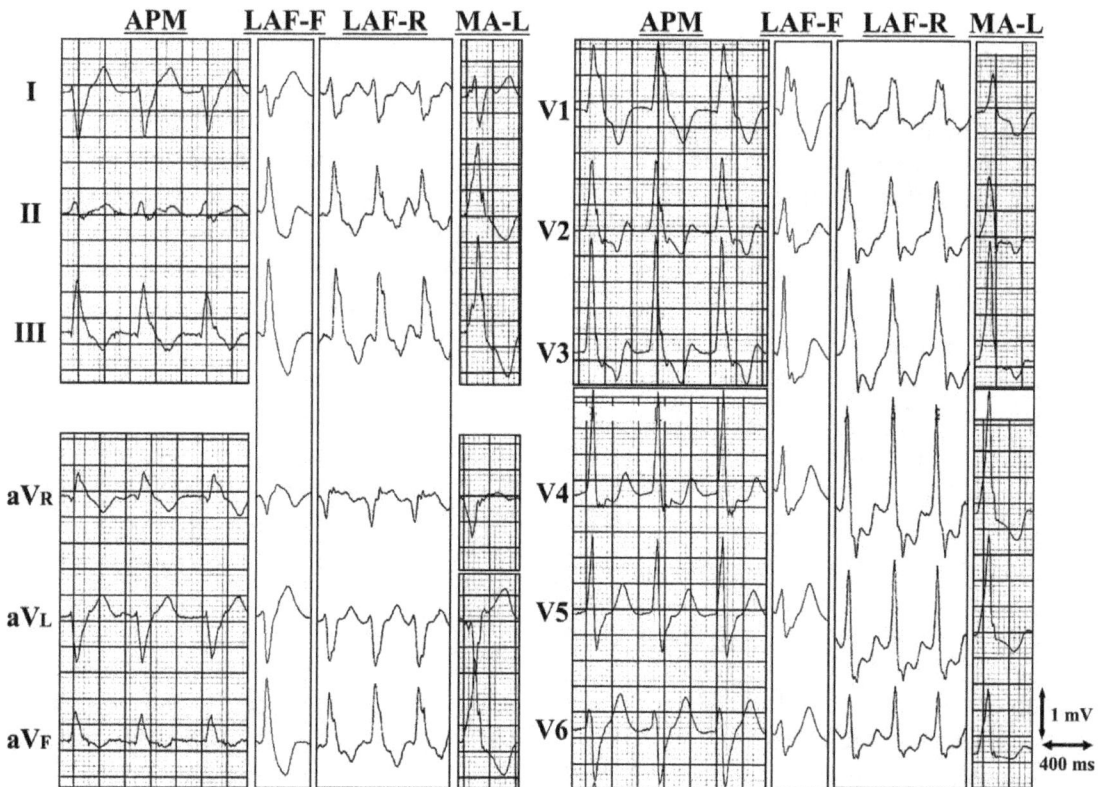

Figure 8. Representative 12-lead electrocardiograms of the QRS complexes during ventricular arrhythmias originating from the anterolateral region in the LV. APM, anterolateral papillary muscle; L, lateral portion; LAF, the left anterior fascicle; MA, mitral annulus; X-F, R, VAs with a focal or a macroreentrant mechanism. This figure was reproduced from Ref. [21] with permission.

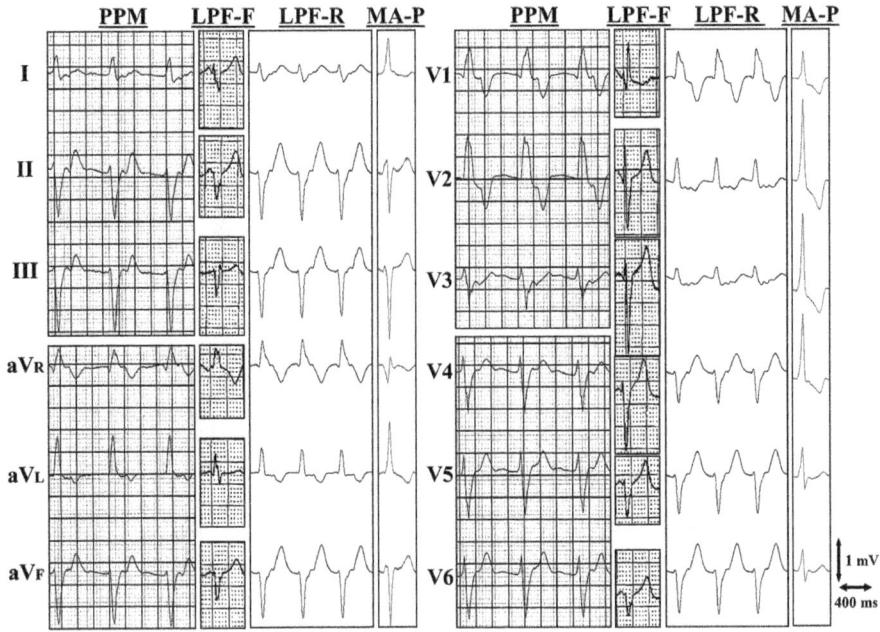

Figure 9. Representative 12-lead electrocardiograms of the QRS complexes during ventricular arrhythmias originating from the posteroseptal region in the LV. LPF, the left posterior fascicle; MA, mitral annulus; P, posterior portion; PPM, posteromedial papillary muscle; X-F, R, VAs with a focal or a macroreentrant mechanism. This figure was reproduced from Ref. [21] with permission.

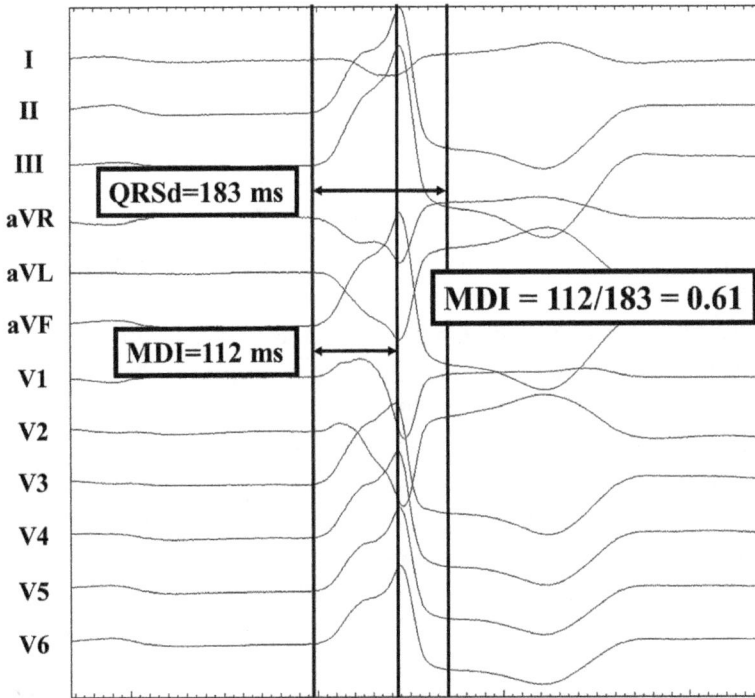

Figure 10. Twelve-lead electrocardiograms exhibiting a ventricular arrhythmia originating from the LV summit and the measurement of the maximal deflection index (MDI). This figure was cited from Ref. [3] with permission.

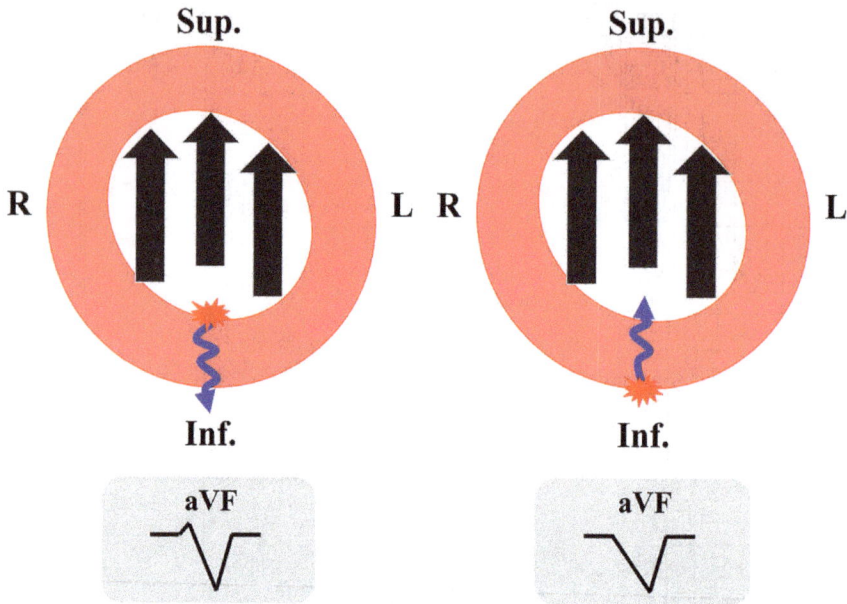

Figure 11. Schema showing the mechanism to explain the difference in the QRS morphology in lead aVF during ventricular tachycardias with endocardial (left) and epicardial (right) foci. Inf, inferior; L, left; R, right; Sup, superior. This figure was cited from Ref. [32] with permission.

endocardial origin on the LV free wall or ventricular posterior wall, a part of the activation vector should go toward the lateral or the inferior direction, which reflects the activation conducting through the wall of the ventricular muscle toward the epicardium, resulting in the presence of an initial R wave in lead I or lead aVF (**Figure 11**). Therefore, a QS pattern in lead I or aVF suggests an epicardial origin in the LV free wall [10] or the ventricular posterior wall, respectively (**Figure 11**). All these ECG features are more accurate without SHD than with it, because without any scar tissue associated with SHD, the ventricular activation propagates away from VA origins through normal ventricular myocardium in a predictable manner.

IVAs originating from the RVOT and LVOT exhibit similar ECG characteristics because anatomically, the RVOT and LVOT are located next to each other (**Figure 3**). The ECGs of idiopathic outflow tract VAs are characterized by positive R waves in all inferior leads and deep S waves in both leads aVR and aVL (almost QS pattern) (**Figures 12–14**). An RBBB QRS morphology clearly suggests a VA origin on the left side. However, when idiopathic outflow tract VAs exhibit an LBBB QRS morphology, it is often difficult to differentiate RVOT VAs from LVOT VAs. Because anatomically, the LVOT is located posterior to the RVOT (**Figure 3**), LVOT VAs exhibit taller and wider R waves in leads V1 and V2 than RVOT VAs. Therefore, the precordial transition is helpful for differentiating RVOT VAs from LVOT VAs. When the precordial transition is later than lead V4, the VAs are very likely to originate from the RVOT, and when the precordial transition is earlier than lead V2, the VAs are very likely to originate from the LVOT. However, when the precordial transition is in lead V3, it is most difficult to differentiate RVOT VAs from LVOT VAs. Although multiple ECG algorithms to differentiate RVOT VAs from LVOT VAs have been proposed, two ECG algorithms may be recommended, the magnitude and width of the R wave or QRS complex in leads V1 and V2

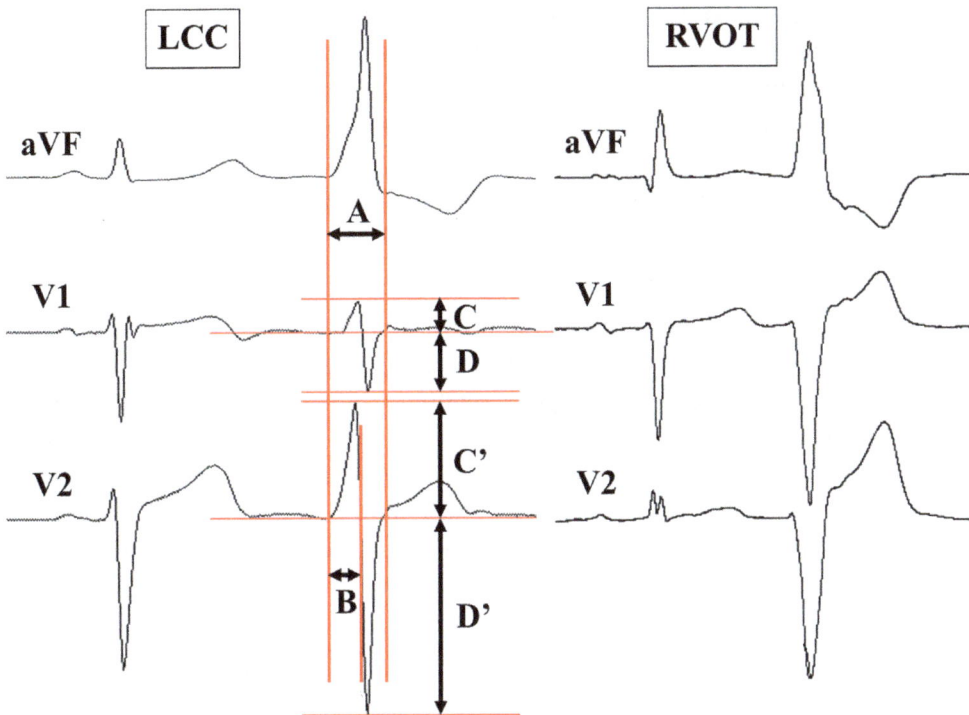

Figure 12. Examples of an electrocardiographic analysis of ventricular arrhythmias. The first beats are sinus and the second beats are ventricular arrhythmias originating from the left coronary cusp (LCC) and the right ventricular outflow tract (RVOT). **A** indicates the total QRS duration, **B** the longer R-wave duration in lead V1 or V2, determined in lead V2 from the QRS onset to the R-wave intersection point where the R-wave crosses the isoelectric line, **C** the R-wave amplitude, measured from the peak to the isoelectric line, and **D** the S-wave amplitude measured from the QRS nadir to the isoelectric line. The R/S wave amplitude ratio in lead V2 (C′/D′) is greater than that in lead V1 (C/D), and C′/D′ is determined as the R/S wave amplitude index. The R/S amplitude index is less than 0.3 and the R-wave duration index (B/A) less than 0.5 during RVOT VAs, whereas they are not during LCC VAs. This figure was cited from Ref. [6] with permission.

(R/S wave amplitude and duration indexes) [8] (**Figure 12**) and V2S/V3R amplitude ratio [35] (**Figure 13**), because they can simply and accurately perform a diagnosis by an ECG of VA only. The R/S wave amplitude in leads V1 and V2 is measured as the amplitude of the QRS complex peak or nadir to the isoelectric line. The R/S wave amplitude index, calculated from the percentage of the R/S wave amplitude ratio in lead V1 or V2 (whichever is greater), is considered more useful than the R/S wave amplitude ratio alone in lead V1 or V2. The R-wave duration index is calculated by dividing the longer R-wave duration in lead V1 or V2 by the QRS complex duration. An R/S amplitude index of <0.3 and an R-wave duration index of <0.5 may strongly suggest a VA origin on the right side (**Figure 13**) [8]. The V2S/V3R amplitude ratio is calculated by dividing the amplitude of the S wave in lead V2 by that of R wave in lead V3. A V2S/V3R amplitude ratio of ≤1.5 can predict LVOT VA origins and that of >1.5 RVOT VA origins (**Figure 13**) [35]. This ECG algorithm is useful even when the precordial transition is observed in lead V3 and has been proven to be the most accurate among the previous ECG algorithms to differentiate RVOT VA origins from LVOT VA origins.

Although the three ASCs are located next to each other, IVAs that can be ablated within each ASC may be differentiated by ECGs (**Figure 14**) [7]. IVAs that can be ablated within the RCC and at the L-RCC rarely exhibit an RBBB pattern, and IVAs that can be ablated within the NCC always exhibit an LBBB pattern. The R-wave amplitude ratio in leads III–II (III/II ratio) is useful for differentiating LCC VAs from RCC VAs. When the III/II ratio is >0.9, VAs are more likely to be ablated within the LCC. A qrS pattern in the right precordial leads may be highly specific for an L-RCC VA origin (**Figure 14**) [13]. The ECG characteristics of NCC VAs are similar to those of RCC VAs (**Figure 14**) [14]. However, an S wave in lead III is present during NCC VAs although it is not during RCC VAs. When the III/II ratio is <0.65, VAs are more likely to be ablated from within the NCC.

All MA VAs exhibit an RBBB pattern and monophasic R or Rs in leads V2–V6 (**Figure 15**) [9, 10]. Because the origins of all MA VAs are located in the posterior portion of the LV, which is distant from the precordial electrodes, the activation from the MA VA origins propagates toward these electrodes, resulting in an early precordial transition and a concordant positive QRS pattern in leads V2–V4 during MA VAs. The ECG characteristics are very helpful for predicting sites of MA VA origins [9, 10]. The polarity of the QRS complex in the inferior and lateral leads (I and aVL) is positive and negative in anterolateral MA VAs, while it is negative

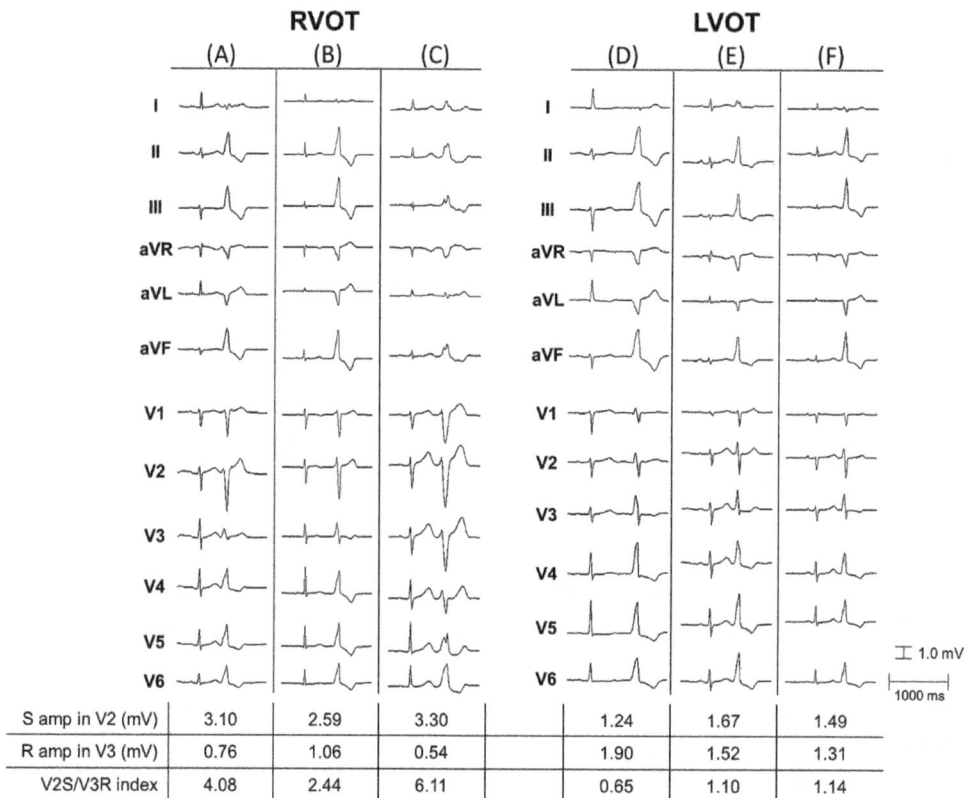

	RVOT				LVOT		
	(A)	(B)	(C)		(D)	(E)	(F)
S amp in V2 (mV)	3.10	2.59	3.30		1.24	1.67	1.49
R amp in V3 (mV)	0.76	1.06	0.54		1.90	1.52	1.31
V2S/V3R index	4.08	2.44	6.11		0.65	1.10	1.14

Figure 13. Representative 12-lead electrocardiograms of VAs originating from the ventricular outflow tract. The first beat is a sinus beat and the second is a premature ventricular contraction in each panel (A–F). The S-wave amplitude in lead V2, R-wave amplitude in lead V3, and V2S/V3R index are listed below each panel. All right ventricular outflow tract (RVOT) PVCs exhibited a V2S/V3R index of >1.5, while all left ventricular outflow tract (LVOT) PVCs exhibited a V2S/V3R index of ≤1.5. The PVCs were successfully ablated in the RVOT septum (A and B), RVOT free wall (C), left coronary cusp (D), right coronary cusp (E), and aorto-mitral continuity (F). The other abbreviation is as in the previous figure. This figure was cited from Ref. [35] with permission.

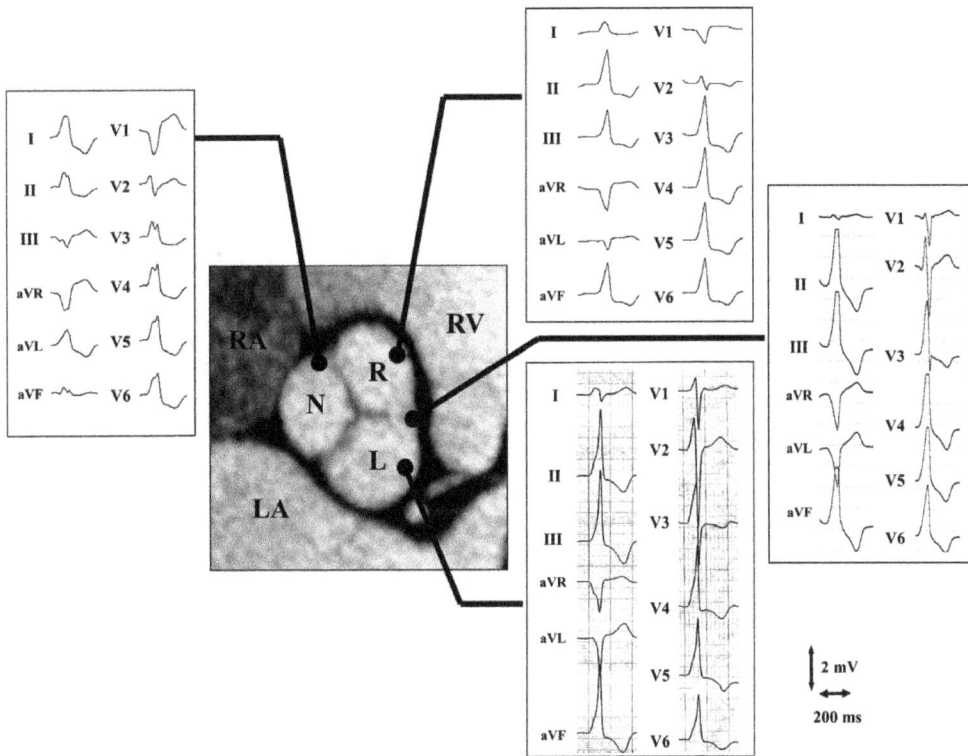

Figure 14. Two-dimensional CT images and representative 12-lead electrocardiograms of ventricular arrhythmias originating from the aortic root. L, left coronary cusp; N, noncoronary cusp; R, right coronary cusp. The other abbreviations are as in the previous figures. This figure was cited from Ref. [7] with permission.

and positive in posterior and posterolateral MA VAs, respectively. MA VAs originating from the free wall of the MA are characterized by a longer QRS duration sometimes with pseudo-delta waves and notching in the late phase of the R or Q wave in the inferior leads, which may result from phased excitation from the LV free wall to the RV (**Figure 15**). Posterior MA VAs exhibit a dominant R wave in lead V1, whereas posteroseptal MA VAs exhibit a negative QRS component in lead V1 (qR, qr, rs, rS, or QS).

All TA VAs exhibit an LBBB QRS morphology and positive QRS polarity in leads I, V5, and V6 (**Figure 16**) [17] because the TA VA origins are located on the right anterior side of the heart, and the activation propagating from TA VA origins toward the apex generates a positive QRS polarity in leads V5 and V6. The R wave in lead I is usually taller during TA VAs than during RVOT VAs because the TA is located more rightward and inferior to the RVOT. For the same reason, a positive QRS polarity in all of the inferior leads is rare in TA VAs but common in all RVOT VAs. During TA VAs, a QS or an rS pattern in lead aVL is rare, and the QRS polarity in lead aVL is positive in almost all TA VAs, which is not the case for RVOT VAs. Among all TA VAs, the QRS duration and Q wave amplitude in each of the leads V1–V3 are greater in TA VAs originating from the free wall of the TA than in those from the septal wall of the TA [17]. Septal TA VAs exhibit an early precordial transition (lead V3), a narrower QRS duration, and QS in lead V1 with the absence of notching in the inferior leads while the free wall TA VAs are associated with a late precordial transition (>lead V3), a wider QRS duration, the absence of Q

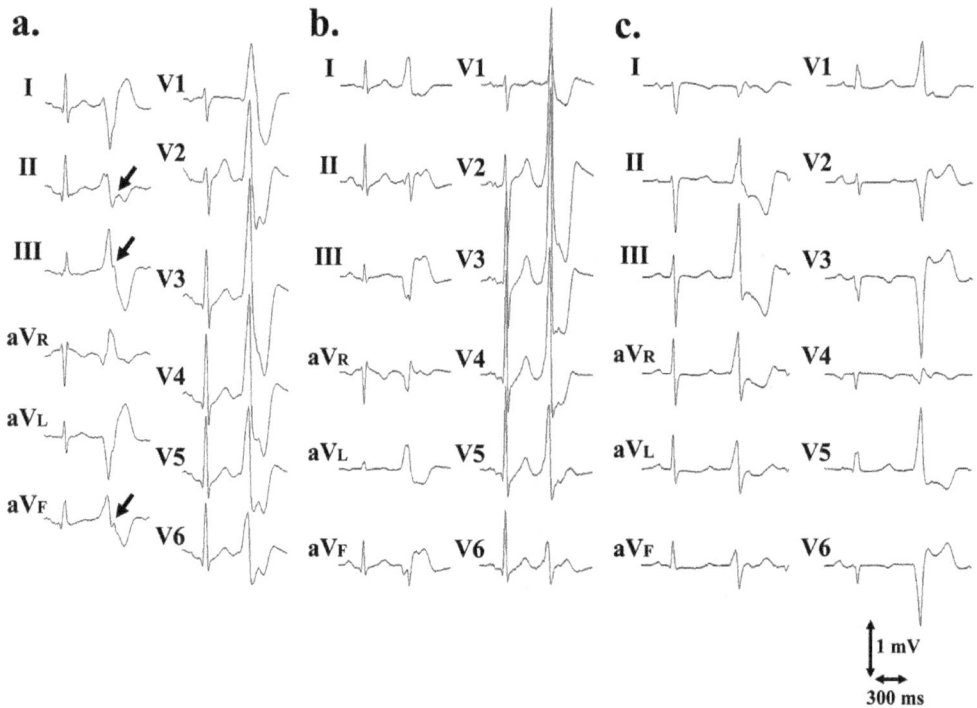

Figure 15. Representative 12-lead electrocardiograms of the premature ventricular contractions originating from the anterolateral (a), posterior (b), and posteroseptal (c) aspects of the mitral annulus. The arrows indicate "notching" of the late phase of the QRS complex in the inferior leads. This figure was cited from Ref. [10] with permission.

waves in lead V1, and the presence of notching in the inferior leads (the timing of the second peak of the notched QRS complex in the inferior leads corresponds precisely with the LV free wall activation) (**Figure 16**). A negative QRS polarity in the inferior leads predicts VA origins in the posterior aspect of the TA, and otherwise, VA origins in the mid- to anterior aspects of the TA are suggested.

IVAs originating from the anterolateral and posteromedial PAMs in the LV exhibit RBBB and right inferior and left or right superior axis QRS morphologies, respectively (**Figures 8 and 9**) [18–21]. IVAs originating from the posterior or anterior RV PAMs more often exhibit a superior axis with a late precordial transition (>lead V4) as compared with septal RV PAM VAs, which more often exhibit an inferior axis with an earlier precordial transition (≤lead V4) [22].

Because of the close anatomical relationship, it is important to distinguish PAM VAs from MA VAs and LV fascicular VAs by ECGs (**Figures 8 and 9**) [21]. The ECG features such as an rS in lead I, an rS in lead aVR (for only the LV anterolateral region), a qR in lead aVL, a Q in lead V1, an S wave amplitude ratio in leads III to II <1.5, and an R/S ratio of ≤1 in lead V6 (the last two parameters are for only the LV posteroseptal region) can accurately distinguish MA VAs from PAM and LV fascicular VAs [21]. However, the ECG features are very similar for PAM and LV fascicular VAs, and an R/S ratio of ≤1 in lead V6 in the LV anterolateral region and a QRS duration of >160 ms, and qR or R waves in lead V1 (as compared with an rsR' for fascicular VTs) in the LV posteroseptal region may be the only reliable predictors for differentiating PAM VAs from LV fascicular VAs [21].

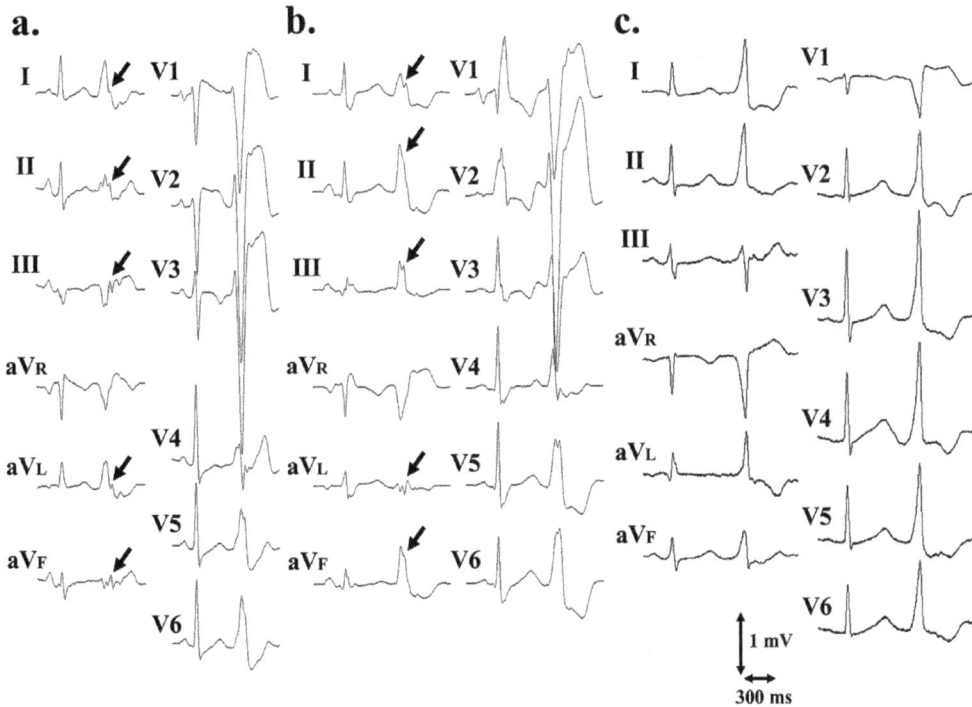

Figure 16. Representative 12-lead electrocardiograms of the premature ventricular contractions originating from the posterolateral (a), anterior (b), and anteroseptal (c) aspects of the tricuspid annulus. The arrows indicate "notching" of the late phase of the QRS complex in the limb leads. This figure was cited from Ref. [10] with permission.

IVAs arising from the MB exhibit a distinctive ECG morphology, LBBB and left superior axis QRS morphology, a sharp downstroke of the QRS in the precordial leads, and a relatively narrow QRS duration (**Figure 4**) [23]. MB VAs not only have a late precordial transition pattern, typically after lead V4, but also the transition is always later than that of the sinus QRS. Among the idiopathic RV VAs, a late precordial transition and a superiorly directed nature are helpful for distinguishing MB VAs from VAs originating from the RV base or septum [23]. The ECG characteristics of the IVAs originating from the infundibular muscles are similar to those of IVAs originating from the RVOT and the anterior to anteroseptal aspect of the TA [24, 25]. However, the precordial transition is relatively early, and a slow onset of the QRS complex is often observed.

IVAs arising from the crux of the heart exhibit a left superior axis QRS morphology with deeply negative deltoid waves (QS pattern) in the inferior leads and an early precordial transition (a prominent R wave in lead V2), which may be associated with a polarity reversal between leads V1 and V2 (**Figure 6**) [30]. It is noted that crux VAs often exhibit a QS or a large S wave in lead V6 although they arise from the LV base. This is likely because the activation from the crux VA origins first conducts to the ventricular apex where it enters the Purkinje system and then propagates throughout the ventricles. The common ECG characteristics of LV summit VAs are a right inferior axis QRS morphology, a wider QRS, and a larger MDI than the other idiopathic LVOT VAs [31]. The MDI [34] of these epicardial IVAs is usually >0.55. The AMC and LV summit face each other with the superior end of the LV muscle between them, which is attached to the LCC. Because of the anatomical proximity, the presence of preferential conduction, and the presence of intramural VA origins, it is challenging to predict where LVOT VAs can be ablated among those three sites by an ECG algorithm [28, 29].

4. Treatment of IVAs

Treatment of IVAs should be tailored according to the presentation type of VAs, PVCs, or VTs, and the patient characteristics (**Figure 17**) [4, 5]. When SHD is absent, the most common indication for treating PVCs remains the presence of symptoms. The severity of the symptoms from PVCs is not closely related to the frequency of PVCs. Even when the PVCs are infrequent, some patients are very symptomatic. When PVCs are not frequent, the physician has to explain and reassure that there is a benign nature of idiopathic PVCs. It is a common experience that symptoms from PVCs can improve without any treatment in most patients with infrequent PVCs. Exercise stress testing should be considered to determine whether PVCs are potentiated or suppressed by exercise, to assess whether longer duration VAs are provoked especially when symptoms are associated with exercise. PVCs that worsen with exercise should prompt further investigation as these patients are more likely to require treatment. Frequent asymptomatic PVCs may have to be treated if PVC-induced cardiomyopathy

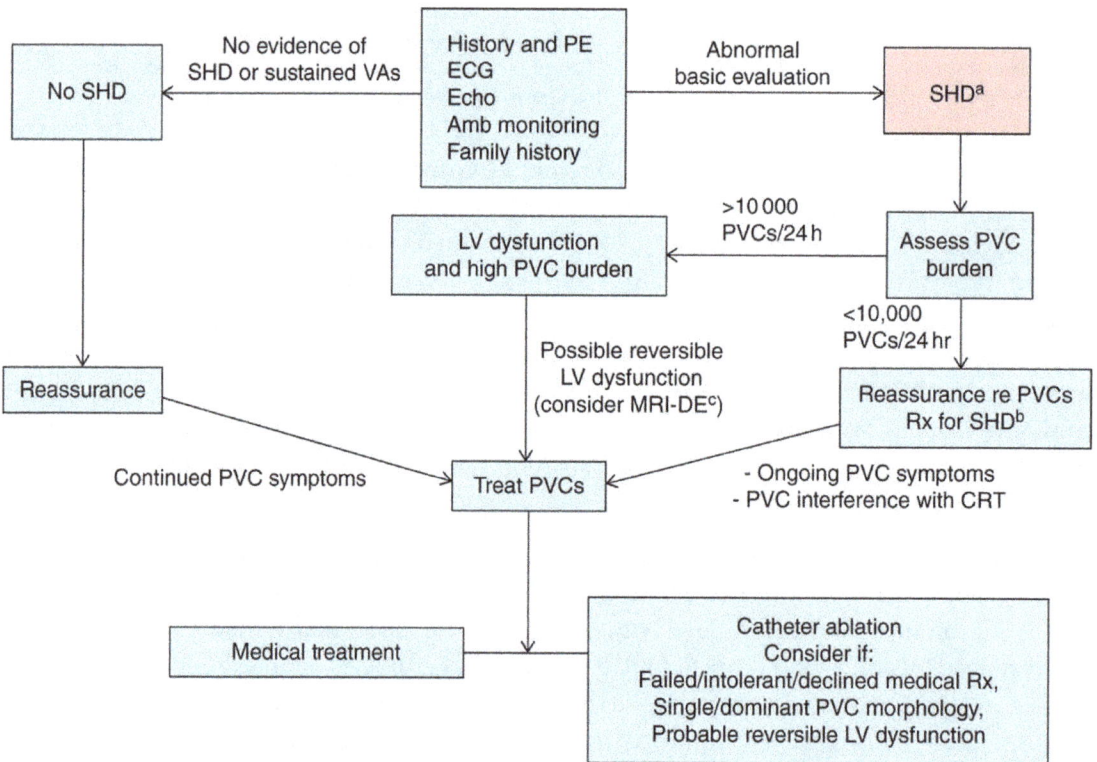

Figure 17. Schema exhibiting the management of premature ventricular contractions (PVCs). (a) Absence of a high-scar burden suggests reversibility; (b) medical therapy + implantable cardioverter-defibrillator. CRT, cardiac resynchronization therapy; LV, left ventricular; MRI-DE, magnetic resonance imaging with delayed enhancement; PE, physical examination; Rx, therapy; SHD, structural heart disease; VAs, ventricular arrhythmias. This figure was cited from Ref. [5] with permission.

is present. When a PVC burden is greater than 10% (approximately 10,000 PVCs/24 h), the risk of PVC-induced cardiomyopathy is significant. Therefore, such high-burdened PVCs have to be treated when they are symptomatic. When they are asymptomatic, a close follow-up with repeat echocardiography and Holter monitoring should be considered to detect any occurrence of PVC-induced cardiomyopathy. In patients with fewer PVCs, further investigation is only necessary should the symptoms increase. For patients without SHD and mild symptoms, education of the benign nature of this arrhythmia and reassurance should be considered as the first step in the treatment of patients with PVCs. For patients whose symptoms are not effectively managed in this manner, beta-blockers or non-dihydropyridine calcium antagonists may be attempted although the efficacy of these agents is quite limited with only 10–15% of patients achieving a 90% PVC suppression, similar to placebo [4, 5]. It should also be recognized that these agents may themselves produce significant side effects rather than relieve the PVC symptoms. Membrane-active anti-arrhythmic drugs (AADs) are more effective for suppressing PVCs and can be attempted when beta-blockers or non-dihydropyridine calcium antagonists are not effective. Because these agents may increase the risk of mortality in patients with significant SHD, perhaps with the exception of amiodarone, caution is advised before using them for PVC suppression.

When idiopathic PVCs are refractory to medication or patients cannot tolerate medication, catheter ablation can be a next option for their treatment. Randomized trials of PVC suppression with catheter ablation have not been performed. However, multiple studies have revealed that catheter ablation is highly successful with PVC elimination in 74–100% of highly symptomatic patients with a very high PVC burden [4, 5]. Procedural success may be dependent on the site of the VA origin with a lower efficacy reported for IVAs with epicardial foci and anatomical challenges than for other IVAs [1–5]. Although complete PVC elimination is the goal of ablation, partial success with a significant reduction in the PVC burden may still be associated with significant improvement in the symptoms as well as LV systolic function. Catheter ablation of IVAs may be less successful when multiple morphologies of PVCs present or the clinical PVC morphology cannot be induced at the time of the procedure [1–5]. The published complication rates of catheter ablation for PVC suppression are generally low (<1%) [1–5]. According to the current recommendations of the experts' consensus, catheter ablation of PVCs may be considered for highly selected patients who remain very symptomatic despite conservative treatment or for those with high PVC burdens associated with a decline in the LV systolic function [4, 5].

Idiopathic VTs are basically monomorphic and hemodynamically stable. When SHD is absent, sustained idiopathic VTs are generally associated with an excellent prognosis [1, 4, 5]. Idiopathic VTs rarely can have a malignant clinical course, usually with a very rapid rate or a short initiating coupling interval [1, 4, 5]. Idiopathic non-sustained VTs (NSVTs) usually present with frequent PVCs with the same QRS morphology, and most of them originate from the RVOT or LVOT. These arrhythmias only require treatment if they are symptomatic, incessant, or produce LV dysfunction. The treatment of these VTs is either medical with beta-blockers, non-hydropyridine calcium blockers, or class IC drugs, or catheter ablation with a high success rate and low risk of complications [1, 4, 5]. Non-sustained and sustained VTs with a focal mechanism likely based on abnormal automaticity may also occur from the papillary muscles and respond to beta-blockers or catheter ablation with a relatively low success rate [4, 5, 18–21]. Reentrant LV fascicular VTs usually present as a sustained form and can be acutely treated with intravenous verapamil or mexiletine. Oral therapy with these medicines can be used to prevent recurrence of those VTs, although the recurrence risk may be relatively high [4, 5, 26, 27]. Catheter ablation can be recommended when idiopathic VTs are highly symptomatic and drug-refractory, especially if they are exercise-induced [1, 4, 5].

Catheter ablation of IVAs is usually safe and highly successful, but sometimes can be challenging because of the anatomical obstacles such as close proximity to the coronary arteries and AV conduction system, epicardial fat pads, intramural and epicardial origins, and thick muscle bands. Understanding the relevant anatomy is helpful for achieving a safe and successful catheter ablation of IVAs.

5. Conclusions

The sites of IVA origins have been increasingly recognized for the past two decades. IVAs usually originate from specific anatomical structures, commonly endocardial but sometimes epicardial, and exhibit characteristic ECGs based on their anatomical background. IVAs are basically benign, but they require medical treatment or catheter ablation when IVAs are symptomatic, incessant, or produce LV dysfunction.

Conflict of interest

The author declares no conflicts of interest.

Author details

Takumi Yamada

Address all correspondence to: takumi-y@fb4.so-net.ne.jp

Division of Cardiovascular Disease, University of Alabama at Birmingham, Birmingham, AL, USA

References

[1] Stevenson WG, Soejima K. Catheter ablation for ventricular tachycardia. Circulation. 2007;**115**:2750-2760

[2] Yamada T, Kay GN. Optimal ablation strategies for different types of ventricular tachycardias. Nature Reviews. Cardiology. 2012;**9**:512-525

[3]   Yamada T. Idiopathic ventricular arrhythmias: Relevance to the anatomy, diagnosis and treatment. Journal of Cardiology. 2016;**68**:463-471

[4]   Pedersen CT, Kay GN, Kalman J, Borggrefe M, Della-Bella P, Dickfeld T, Dorian P, Huikuri H, Kim YH, Knight B, Marchlinski F, Ross D, Sacher F, Sapp J, Shivkumar K, Soejima K, Tada H, Alexander ME, Triedman JK, Yamada T, Kirchhof P, Document Reviewers, Lip GY, Kuck KH, Mont L, Haines D, Indik J, Dimarco J, Exner D, Iesaka Y, Savelieva I. EHRA/HRS/APHRS expert consensus on ventricular arrhythmias. Europace. 2014;**16**:1257-1283

[5]   Pedersen CT, Kay GN, Kalman J, Borggrefe M, Della-Bella P, Dickfeld T, Dorian P, Huikuri H, Kim YH, Knight B, Marchlinski F, Ross D, Sacher F, Sapp J, Shivkumar K, Soejima K, Tada H, Alexander ME, Triedman JK, Yamada T, Kirchhof P, Lip GY, Kuck KH, Mont L, Haines D, Indik J, Dimarco J, Exner D, Iesaka Y, Savelieva I, EP-Europace, UK. EHRA/HRS/APHRS expert consensus on ventricular arrhythmias. Heart Rhythm. 2014;**11**:e166-e196

[6]   Yamada T, Kay GN. How to diagnose and ablate ventricular tachycardia from the outflow tract and aortic cusps. In: Al-Ahmad A, Callans DJ, Hsia HH, Natale A, Oseroff O, Wang PJ, editors. Hands-On Ablation: The Experts' Approach. 2nd ed. Minneapolis, MN: Cardiotext Publishing; 2017. pp. 292-301

[7]   Yamada T, McElderry HT, Doppalapudi H, Murakami Y, Yoshida Y, Yoshida N, Okada T, Tsuboi N, Inden Y, Murohara T, Epstein AE, Plumb VJ, Singh SP, Kay GN. Idiopathic ventricular arrhythmias originating from the aortic root: Prevalence, electrocardiographic and electrophysiological characteristics, and results of the radiofrequency catheter ablation. Journal of the American College of Cardiology. 2008;**52**:139-147

[8]   Ouyang F, Fotuhi P, Ho SY, Hebe J, Volkmer M, Goya M, Burns M, Antz M, Ernst S, Cappato R, Kuck KH. Repetitive monomorphic ventricular tachycardia originating from the aortic sinus cusp: Electrocardiographic characterization for guiding catheter ablation. Journal of the American College of Cardiology. 2002;**39**:500-508

[9]   Tada H, Ito S, Naito S, Kurosaki K, Kubota S, Sugiyasu A, Tsuchiya T, Miyaji K, Yamada M, Kutsumi Y, Oshima S, Nogami A, Taniguchi K. Idiopathic ventricular arrhythmia arising from the mitral annulus: A distinct subgroup of idiopathic ventricular arrhythmias. Journal of the American College of Cardiology. 2005;**45**:877-886

[10] Yamada T. Idiopathic ventricular tachycardia from mitral annulus, papillary muscles and other sites. In: Bhargava K, Asirvatham SJ. Practical Cardiac Electrophysiology. Jaypee Brothers Medical Publishers Pvt. Ltd.; 2016. pp. 543-66

[11] McAlpine WA. Heart and Coronary Arteries. New York: Springer-Verlag; 1975

[12] Yamada T, Litovsky SH, Kay GN. The left ventricular ostium: An anatomic concept relevant to idiopathic ventricular arrhythmias. Circulation. Arrhythmia and Electrophysiology. 2008;**1**:396-404

[13] Yamada T, Yoshida N, Murakami Y, Okada T, Muto M, Murohara T, McElderry HT, Kay GN. Electrocardiographic characteristics of ventricular arrhythmias originating from the

junction of the left and right coronary sinuses of Valsalva in the aorta: The activation pattern as a rationale for the electrocardiographic characteristics. Heart Rhythm. 2008;5:184-192

[14] Yamada T, Lau YR, Litovsky SH, Thomas McElderry H, Doppalapudi H, Osorio J, Plumb VJ, Neal Kay G. Prevalence and clinical, electrocardiographic, and electrophysiologic characteristics of ventricular arrhythmias originating from the noncoronary sinus of Valsalva. Heart Rhythm. 2013;10:1605-1612

[15] Yamada T, McElderry HT, Doppalapudi H, Kay GN. Catheter ablation of ventricular arrhythmias originating in the vicinity of the His bundle: Significance of mapping the aortic sinus cusp. Heart Rhythm. 2008;5:37-42

[16] Sekiguchi Y, Aonuma K, Takahashi A, Yamauchi Y, Hachiya H, Yokoyama Y, Iesaka Y, Isobe M. Electrocardiographic and electrophysiologic characteristics of ventricular tachycardia originating within the pulmonary artery. Journal of the American College of Cardiology. 2005;45:887-895

[17] Tada H, Tadokoro K, Ito S, Naito S, Hashimoto T, Kaseno K, Miyaji K, Sugiyasu A, Tsuchiya T, Kutsumi Y, Nogami A, Oshima S, Taniguchi K. Idiopathic ventricular arrhythmias originating from the tricuspid annulus: Prevalence, electrocardiographic characteristics, and results of radiofrequency catheter ablation. Heart Rhythm. 2007;4:7-16

[18] Doppalapudi H, Yamada T, McElderry HT, Plumb VJ, Epstein AE, Kay GN. Ventricular tachycardia originating from the posterior papillary muscle in the left ventricle: A distinct clinical syndrome. Circulation. Arrhythmia and Electrophysiology. 2008;1:23-29

[19] Yamada T, McElderry HT, Okada T, Murakami Y, Doppalapudi H, Yoshida N, Allred JD, Murohara T, Kay GN. Idiopathic focal ventricular arrhythmias originating from the anterior papillary muscle in the left ventricle. Journal of Cardiovascular Electrophysiology. 2009;20:866-872

[20] Yamada T, Doppalapudi H, McElderry HT, Okada T, Murakami Y, Inden Y, Yoshida Y, Yoshida N, Murohara T, Epstein AE, Plumb VJ, Litovsky SH, Kay GN. Electrocardiographic and electrophysiological characteristics in idiopathic ventricular arrhythmias originating from the papillary muscles in the left ventricle: Relevance for catheter ablation. Circulation. Arrhythmia and Electrophysiology. 2010;3:324-331

[21] Yamada T, Doppalapudi H, McElderry HT, Okada T, Murakami Y, Inden Y, Yoshida Y, Kaneko S, Yoshida N, Murohara T, Epstein AE, Plumb VJ, Kay GN. Idiopathic ventricular arrhythmias originating from the papillary muscles in the left ventricle: Prevalence, electrocardiographic and electrophysiological characteristics, and results of the radiofrequency catheter ablation. Journal of Cardiovascular Electrophysiology. 2010;21:62-69

[22] Crawford T, Mueller G, Good E, Jongnarangsin K, Chugh A, Pelosi F Jr, Ebinger M, Oral H, Morady F, Bogun F. Ventricular arrhythmias originating from papillary muscles in the right ventricle. Heart Rhythm. 2010;7:725-730

[23] Sadek MM, Benhayon D, Sureddi R, Chik W, Santangeli P, Supple GE, Hutchinson MD, Bala R, Carballeira L, Zado ES, Patel VV, Callans DJ, Marchlinski FE, Garcia FC. Idiopathic

ventricular arrhythmias originating from the moderator band: Electrocardiographic characteristics and treatment by catheter ablation. Heart Rhythm. 2015;**12**:67-75

[24] Yamada T, Yoshida N, Itoh T, Litovsky SH, Doppalapudi H, McElderry HT, Kay GN. Idiopathic ventricular arrhythmias originating from the parietal band: Electrocardiographic and electrophysiological characteristics and outcome of catheter ablation. Circulation. Arrhythmia and Electrophysiology. 2017;**10**:e005099

[25] Yamada T, Yoshida N, Litovsky SH, Itoh T, Doppalapudi H, Kay GN. Idiopathic ventricular arrhythmias originating from the infundibular muscles: Prevalence, electrocardiographic and electrophysiological characteristics and outcome of catheter ablation. Circulation: Arrhythmia and Electrophysiology. 2018;**11**:e005749

[26] Tsuchiya T, Okumura K, Honda T, Honda T, Iwasa A, Yasue H, Tabuchi T. Significance of late diastolic potential preceding Purkinje potential in verapamil-sensitive idiopathic left ventricular tachycardia. Circulation. 1999;**99**:2408-2413

[27] Nogami A, Naito S, Tada H, Taniguchi K, Okamoto Y, Nishimura S, Yamauchi Y, Aonuma K, Goya M, Iesaka Y, Hiroe M. Demonstration of diastolic and presystolic Purkinje potentials as critical potentials in a macroreentry circuit of verapamil-sensitive idiopathic left ventricular tachycardia. Journal of the American College of Cardiology. 2000;**36**:811-823

[28] Yamada T, Maddox WR, McElderry HT, Doppalapudi H, Plumb VJ, Kay GN. Radiofrequency catheter ablation of idiopathic ventricular arrhythmias originating from intramural foci in the left ventricular outflow tract: Efficacy of sequential versus simultaneous unipolar catheter ablation. Circulation. Arrhythmia and Electrophysiology. 2015;**8**:344-352

[29] Yamada T, Doppalapudi H, Maddox WR, McElderry HT, Plumb VJ, Kay GN. Prevalence and electrocardiographic and electrophysiological characteristics of idiopathic ventricular arrhythmias originating from intramural foci in the left ventricular outflow tract. Circulation: Arrhythmia and Electrophysiology. 2016;**9**:pii: e004079

[30] Doppalapudi H, Yamada T, Ramaswamy K, Ahn J, Kay GN. Idiopathic focal epicardial ventricular tachycardia originating from the crux of the heart. Heart Rhythm. 2009;**6**:44-50

[31] Yamada T, McElderry HT, Doppalapudi H, Okada T, Murakami Y, Yoshida Y, Yoshida N, Inden Y, Murohara T, Plumb VJ, Kay GN. Idiopathic ventricular arrhythmias originating from the left ventricular summit: Anatomic concepts relevant to ablation. Circulation. Arrhythmia and Electrophysiology. 2010;**3**:616-623.0

[32] Yamada T. Transthoracic epicardial catheter ablation: Indications, techniques, and complications. Circulation Journal. 2013;**77**:1672-1680

[33] Berruezo A, Mont L, Nava S, Chueca E, Bartholomay E, Brugada J. Electrocardiographic recognition of the epicardial origin of ventricular tachycardias. Circulation. 2004;**109**: 1842-1847

[34] Daniels DV, Lu YY, Morton JB, Santucci PA, Akar JG, Green A, Wilber DJ. Idiopathic epicardial left ventricular tachycardia originating remote from the sinus of Valsalva: Electrophysiological characteristics, catheter ablation, and identification from the 12-lead electrocardiogram. Circulation. 2006;**113**:1659-1666

[35] Yoshida N, Yamada T, McElderry HT, Inden Y, Shimano M, Murohara T, Kumar V, Doppalapudi H, Plumb VJ, Kay GN. A novel electrocardiographic criterion for differentiating a left from right ventricular outflow tract tachycardia origin: The V2S/V3R index. Journal of Cardiovascular Electrophysiology. 2014;**25**:747-753

9

Surgical Treatment of Atrial Fibrillation

Claudia M. Loardi, Marco Zanobini and
Francesco Alamanni

Abstract

Atrial fibrillation represents the most common supraventricular arrhythmia above all in patients undergoing cardiac surgery and is associated to an augmented risk of thromboembolic stroke, heart failure, and cardiovascular mortality. That is the reason why cardiac surgeons began to address their attention to how to surgically treat fibrillating patients according to pathophysiological models describing mechanisms of arrhythmia induction and maintenance. A new branch of cardiac surgery was born, leading to a progressive development of adapted surgical ablation techniques, applicable both to lone or concomitant arrhythmia treatment. Historical evolution and current available surgical treatment options are described, beginning from the first pure surgical maze, going through all its modifications in source ablation energies and lesion sets and finishing with current mini-invasive hybrid treatment of lone atrial fibrillation. Indications, patients' selection, technical options with respective advantages and disadvantages, surgical technique details, complications, and results are fully illustrated. Relationship between pathophysiologic arrhythmia mechanisms and the consequent ablation tailored procedure choice is highlighted, allowing a customized procedural offer to every single patient, resulting in a success rate ranging from 60 to 90%.

Keywords: atrial fibrillation treatment, maze procedure, hybrid ablation, energy sources, cardiac surgery

1. Introduction

Atrial fibrillation (AF) is a common medical condition affecting over 5 million people in the United States and whose prevalence is expected to join over 12 million by 2030. Considering people aged more than 80 years, about 7% experiences at least one episode of such supraventricular arrhythmia in their life. Dangers of AF are well known; they range from troubling symptoms to a fivefold increased risk of thromboembolic stroke and heart failure and culminate in excess mortality [1]. Cardiac surgeons are frequently faced to AF, since data from the Society of Thoracic Surgeons (STS) database demonstrate that preoperative AF is present in 11% of patients presenting for nonemergent, first-time cardiac surgery, varying from 6.5% of coronary patients until nearly 30% in mitral ones [2]. The high AF prevalence in case of mitral stenosis or regurgitation may be explained by histological modifications occurring in enlarged left atria suggesting chronic inflammation and interstitial fibrosis which translate into electrical changes such as augmentation of effective atrial refractory period and conduction heterogeneity able to lead to an increased vulnerability to arrhythmia genesis. These epidemiologic considerations explain why, historically, cardiac surgeons were the pioneers of curative ablation of AF; their interest began in the 1980s when Cox and associates introduced the left atrial isolation procedure in dogs. A new branch of cardiac surgery was born, leading to a progressive development of adapted surgical ablation sets of lesions and devices, applicable both to lone and concomitant (a term indicating patients in whom AF is associated with another cardiac disease requiring surgery) arrhythmia treatment.

2. Main body

2.1. History: the maze (cut-and-sew procedure)

The history of the surgical treatment of AF began in 1980, when Cox described the procedure of left atrial surgical isolation. This technique was able to enclose arrhythmia in the left atrium, leaving the right one and the ventricle in a synchronized sinusal rhythm (SR). In spite of its hemodynamic efficacy, thromboembolic risk remained unchanged as the left atrium continued to fibrillate. It was clear that the development of a more complete technique was necessary in order to contemporarily achieve SR and atrio-ventricular synchrony maintenance, atrial contractility restoring, and embolic risk elimination. The Cox-maze procedure was introduced in humans in 1987 (called Cox-maze I) developing from results obtained in canine models. It consisted in creating multiple incisions that could block all possible macro-reentrant circuits and direct the propagation of the sinus impulse throughout both atria. Lesions were created by a "cut-and-sew" method performed under direct vision with the advantage of increasing the probability to achieve transmurality. Excision of the left atrial appendage (LAA) was also performed alongside [1]. Even if the goal of freedom from stroke was achieved, occasional left atrial dysfunction and frequent inability to generate adequate sinus tachycardia in response to exercise (chronotrope response) led to the development of the Cox-maze II modification [3]. Sinus node incision was not included in ablation set, and the left atrial upper line was situated more posteriorly. Later, Cox-maze II rapidly evolved and perfected into Cox-maze III, whose ablation schema is represented in **Figure 1**. It consisted in a series of incisions and suture lines in both atria: lines surrounding pulmonary veins orifices with linking lesions between them and with the mitral annulus (isthmus line) and the LAA, both appendages excision and right atrial full set lesions. The Cox-maze III allowed the long-term preservation of atrial transport and sinus node function, decreasing the need for a pacemaker and the recurrence of arrhythmia, while improving the speed of the procedure with requirement of minor technical ability [4].

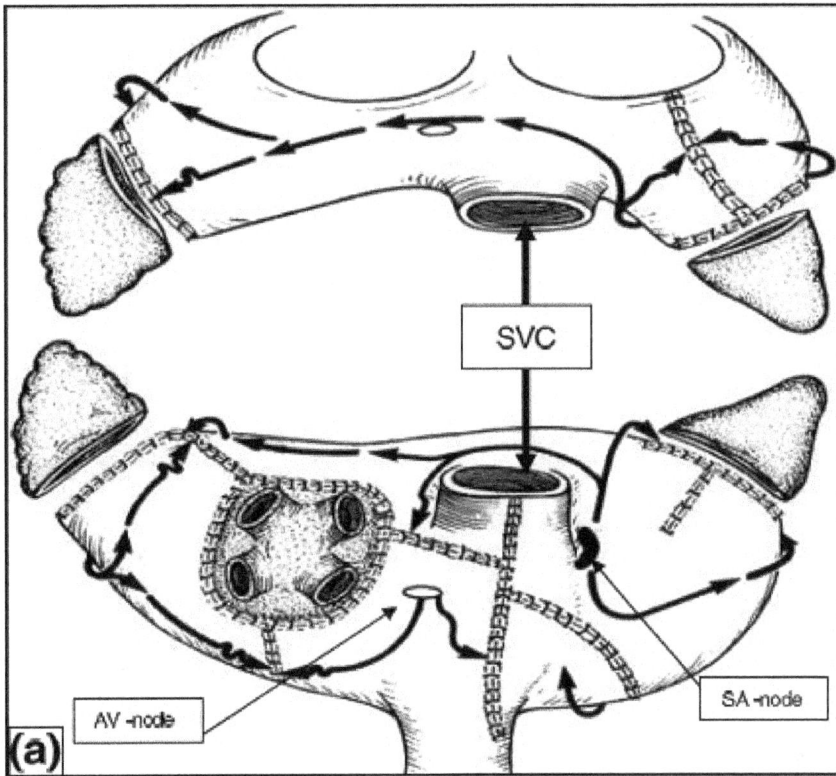

Figure 1. Cox-maze III lesions set.

Cox-maze III showed a proven efficacy with a long-term success rate superior to 90% both in concomitant and in isolated procedures [5]. Nevertheless, other works reported less encouraging results, generating a not unanimous consensus between cardiologists and cardiac surgeons, also partially due to its relevant technical complexity and possible complications. In fact, mortality rate was not irrelevant, since it ranged from 0.7 to 2% and even serious complications were frequently reported (6% following Cox JL and 3.2% in Mayo Clinic experience) including definitive pacemaker implantation due to sinus node injury, stroke, and major bleeding requiring surgical re-exploration.

2.2. Cox-maze evolution

In subsequent years, many attempts were made in order to improve the simplicity of the treatment, evolution which was facilitated by the increasing comprehension of AF patho-physiology thanks to the development of clinic mapping systems. In 1998, Haissaguerre [6] showed that paroxysmal arrhythmia triggers were located at the level of pulmonary veins origin, thus suggesting that an ablation action limited to this zone could be effective. Although the theory of a preeminent role played by pulmonary veins triggers is not applicable to all AF types (for instance, in case of long-standing persistent or permanent AF, other mechanisms are involved in arrhythmia beginning and perpetuating [7]), such discovery paved the way to the trial, by one side, to reduce lesions set by concentrating onto the arrhythmia real sources

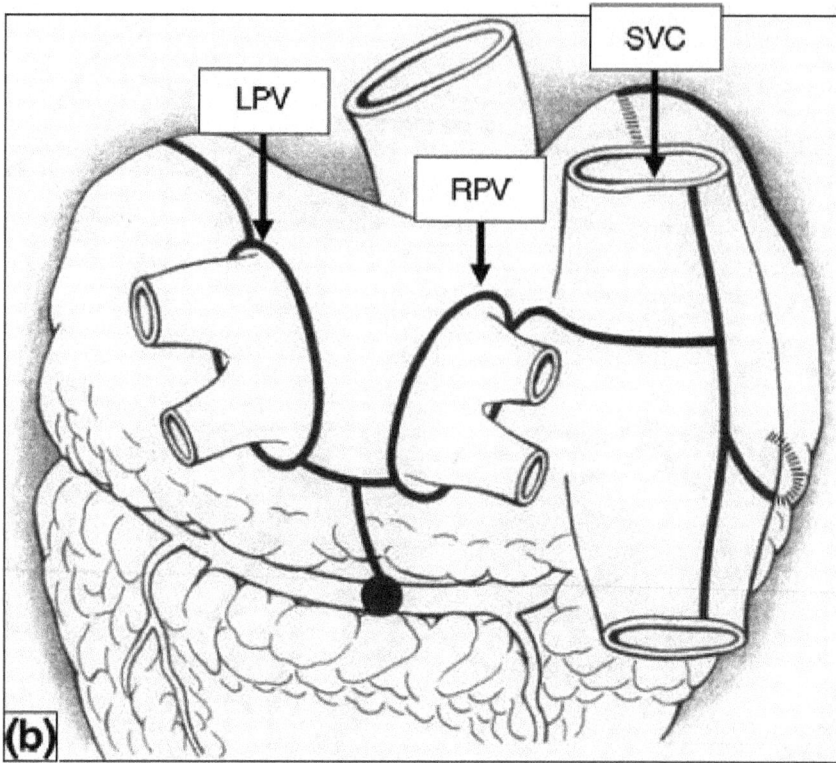

Figure 2. Cox-maze IV lesions set.

and maintaining pathways and, by the other, to minimize surgical risk by replacing lines of incisions by lines of transmural necrosis using other energy sources. In 1999, the first "non cut-and-sew" maze was performed by the use of the cryoenergy as the sole ablation modality for all lesions described in the Cox-maze III; later, Dr. Cox introduced the so-called Cox IV which preserved the entire lesions set of the previous version, but used bipolar radiofrequency (RF) instead of the cut-and-sew technique (**Figure 2**). Minor variations of the ablation procedure have been proposed over time, namely concerning the extension of the lesions set, but the original schema of the Cox-maze IV will remain as the reference for every complete biatrial surgical ablation of long-standing persistent or permanent AF [8].

2.3. Energy sources

2.3.1. Requirements for surgical ablation

In order to perform an effective and durable AF ablation with alternative energy sources replacing surgery, devices and technologies must possess several features [9]:

1. Transmurality: heart lesions, either performed from the epicardial or the endocardial surface, have to go homogeneously through the whole thickness of cardiac wall for producing a complete conduction block with the aim of stopping activation wave fronts or isolating trigger foci. Especially in case of epicardial application on the beating heart, transmurality may be very difficult to achieve due to the heat sink effect of the circulating intracavitary

blood. That is the reason why some energy sources, incapable to overcome such an obstacle, have been quickly abandoned.

2. Safety: excessive or inadequate ablation needs to be avoided by the creation of precise dose–response curves specific for each device. Moreover, energy sources may have different harmful effects onto surrounding vital structures, including coronaries, valves, and esophagus which must be fully known and prevented.

3. Facility and speed: this presupposes that the device must rapidly act and be flexible and easy to handle.

4. Adaptability for minimally invasive approaches: this would require a specific device design allowing its insertion into small thoracotomies or ports.

Over the years, different energy sources have been tested in order to achieve all these requirements [9]: actually, only cryoenergy and radiofrequency (RF) are available and still used, because microwave devices, lasers, and high-frequency ultrasound were progressively abandoned due to their incapacity to produce reliable transmural lesions, thus resulting in high AF recurrence rates. A summary of all energy sources features is shown in **Table 1**.

2.3.2. Anatomic considerations

Human atrial wall thickness is far to be homogeneous in all regions and in every subject [10]; such anatomic consideration plays a major role when a new ablation device performance is tested since it has a direct repercussion onto its ability of creating transmural lesions. In normal individuals, the atrial thickness in the left atrium ranges from 2.3 to 6.5 mm. In patients with any cardiac disease, the mean left atrium thickness is 5.2 ± 1.8 mm. These values encompass muscle thickness only and did not include overlying fat or underlying free-running pectinate muscles, which exist in both atria (which are not continuous with the epicardial surface). In normal individuals, the fat layer at the posterior mitral annulus can be 10-mm thick or more, which is important because epicardial fat can be an obstacle to achieve an adequate depth of penetration for most ablation technologies. Finally, as patients grow older, their chamber size and wall thickness increase. All these anatomic variations and physiologic changes provide a challenge to any unidirectional device to achieve transmural lesions and must be carefully taken into account during ablation procedure.

2.3.3. Cryoablation

Actually, two sources of cryothermal energy are used in cardiac surgery [9]:

1. Nitrous oxide technology (older): its name is cryoICE (AtriCure, Inc., Cincinnati, OH) and uses a 10-cm malleable probe on a 20-cm shaft.

2. Argon technology (Medtronic ATS. Minneapolis, MN): it can be used in two ways, either as a malleable single-use cryosurgical probe with an adjustable insulation sleeve for varying ablation zone lengths or as a two-in-one convertible device that incorporates a clamp and surgical probe (**Figure 3**).

Energy source	Pros	Cons	Application
Cryo	Transmural	Time-consuming	Stand-alone maze, concomitant maze, and lesion subsets Adjunct to RF especially for lesions in perivalvular tissue
Bipolar RF	Transmural Quick Real-time conductance control	Endocardial access need Multiple applications	Stand-alone maze, concomitant maze, and lesion subsets
Unipolar RF	Epi- and endocardial	Low transmurality rates No real-time transmurality control Collateral damage	Stand-alone maze, concomitant maze, and as adjunct with other energy sources
Laser	Quick Epi- and endocardial Good penetration of adipose tissue	No real-time transmurality control Collateral damage	Not currently used
Microwave	Epi- and endocardial	Low transmurality rates Time-consuming No real-time transmurality control Collateral damage	Not currently used
High-intensity focus ultrasound	Epi- and endocardial Defined depth-limiting collateral damage	Time-consuming No real-time transmurality control	Not currently used

Table 1. Comparison of ablation energy sources.

These two devices reach different minimal tissue temperatures (−89.5 and −185.7°C, respectively) but both deliver energy to myocardium by a cryoprobe. In both cases, a console houses the tank containing the liquid refrigerant which is pumped under high pressure to the electrode through an inner lumen. Once the fluid reaches the electrode, it converts from a liquid to a gas phase, absorbing energy and resulting in rapid cooling of the tissue. At the tissue-electrode interface, there is a well-demarcated line of frozen tissue, sometimes termed an "ice ball."

Ablation mechanism consists in cell membrane and cytoplasmatic organelle destruction secondary to the formation of extra- and intracellular ice crystals. In the first 48 h after cryoablation, hemorrhage, edema, inflammation and extending, and irreversible apoptosis occur. Healing is characterized by extensive fibrosis, which begins approximately 1 week after lesion formation.

Cryoablation is unique among the presently available technologies, in that it destroys tissue by freezing instead of heating. The biggest advantage of this technology is its ability to preserve tissue architecture and the collagen structure, making it an excellent energy of source for ablation close to valvular tissue or the fibrous skeleton of the heart.

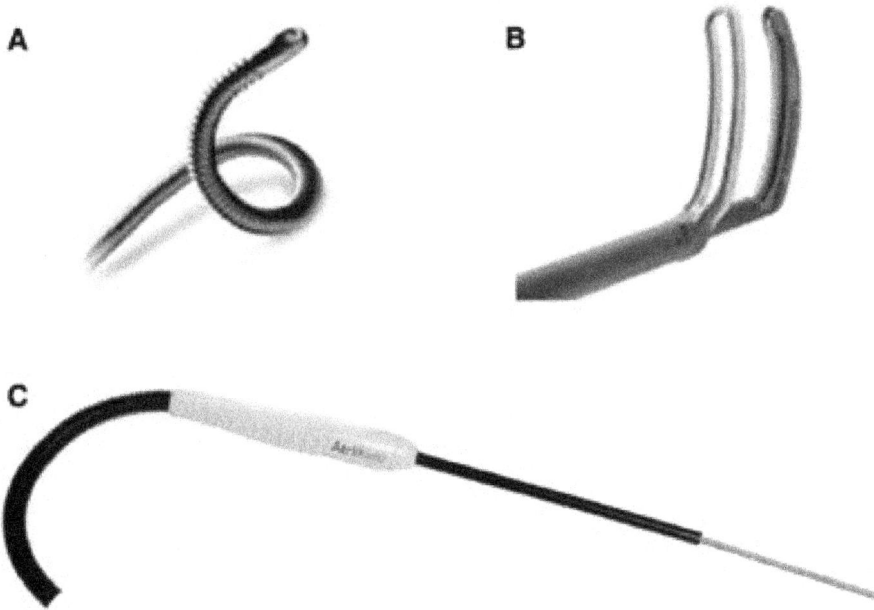

Figure 3. Available devices for cryoablation.

Concerning transmurality and safety profile, nitrous oxide technology provides good performances [11] but may cause injury to coronary arteries. Argon is relatively recent, but it seems to be able to reliably create endocardial safe transmural lesions on the arrested heart. Potential disadvantages of this technology include the relatively long time necessary to create an ablation (2–3 min; **Table 1**) and the detrimental effect of hot circulating blood volume onto cryoenergy when applied in the beating heart without cardioplegic arrest. In order to overcome such problem, a cryoclamp equipped with two arms catching the tissue to be ablated has been recently proposed: in preliminary works, it showed, by one side, a 93% transmurality rate on the beating heart, but, by the other, an increased risk of thromboembolism due to coagulation of the frozen blood.

2.3.4. Unipolar radiofrequency energy

RF energy has been used for cardiac ablation for many years in the electrophysiology laboratory and can be delivered by either unipolar or bipolar electrodes [9].

Several devices are available (**Figure 4**):

1. Estech developed two unipolar surgical probes, the Cobra Adhere XL Probe (Atricure, Inc.) and the Cobra Cooled Surgical Probe (Boston Scientific Corp., Marlborough, MA, USA). These flexible and malleable devices with multiple electrodes, suction system stabilization, and internal saline cooling present the same mode of operation but the second one is specifically designed for minimally invasive approach;

2. VisiTrax (nContact, Raleigh, NC): a coiled electrode that is held in place with suction and irrigated with saline for cooling;

3. Cardioblate Standard Ablation Pen and Cardioblate XL Surgical Ablation Pen by Medtronic: these are pen-like, irrigated unipolar RF devices used to make point-by-point ablations by dragging them across the tissue to make a linear lesion. The Cardioblate XL has a 20-cm shaft and is designed to be used through a port or a small thoracotomy.

RF mode of operation consists in the application of an alternating current in the range of 100–1.000 kHz (high enough to prevent ventricular fibrillation and yet low to prevent tissue perforation) which induces a resistive tissue heating within a narrow rim of <1 mm in direct contact with the electrode and a passive heating in the deeper tissue via conduction. In unipolar technology, a passive electrode must be applied to the patient to allow energy dispersion from the electrode. RF catheters are usually irrigated with saline solutions in order to lower tissue warming and limit scar formation at the interface electrode tissue which greatly limits deep energy penetration and thus ablation efficacy. These irrigated catheters have been shown to create larger volume lesions than dry RF devices [12].

Just after unipolar RF ablation, focal irreversible coagulation necrosis occurs; later, it transforms into contraction and scarring. In case of very high temperature application (>100°C), char formation predominates.

One of the main problems of unipolar RF is its lack of transmurality in a great percentage of cases and this despite long ablation time: more in detail, if on the arrested animal heart transmurality achievement was satisfactory, after 2-min endocardial ablation in humans, only 20% of lesions were transmural and only 7% in case of epicardial application at a temperature of 90°C.

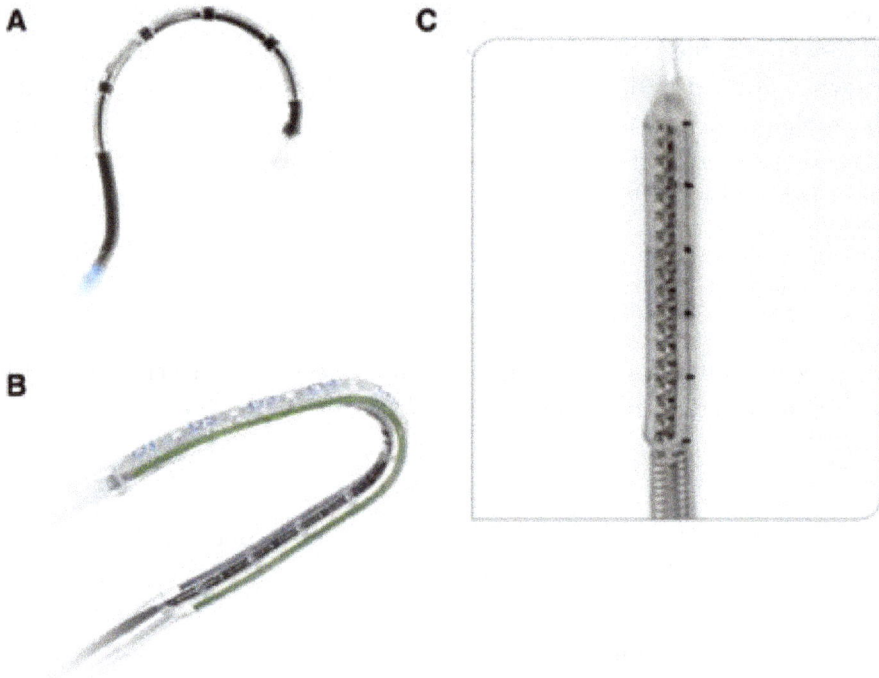

Figure 4. Available devices for unipolar RF ablation.

The complications of unipolar RF devices have been described after extensive clinical use and include coronary artery injuries, cerebrovascular accidents, and the devastating creation of esophageal perforation, leading to atrioesophageal fistula.

2.3.5. Bipolar radiofrequency energy

Bipolar technology is incorporated into devices (**Figure 5**) in two ways [9]:

1. a clamp with two ablating jaws each equipped with electrodes;

2. a device with two side-by-side electrodes applicable both endo- and epicardially.

Various examples of both technologies are commercially available: Atricure Inc., for instance, developed, in the first group, the Isolator Sinergy clamp showing different models and curvatures with a continuous measurement of tissue impedance as a marker of transmurality, or, in the second one, the Isolator Multifunctional Pen able to record electrograms or pacing in addition to ablation function. Atricure has also developed the Coolrail Linear Pen, a 30-mm side-by-side electrode internally cooled with irrigated saline. Both these pens are applied for a fixed period because algorithms assessing transmurality are not available for side-by-side devices.

Medtronic markets three bipolar clamp devices, all with irrigated flexible jaws and an articulating head: the Cardioblate BP2 (arms length of 7 cm), the Cardioblate LP for mini-invasive approach, and the longer Cardioblate Gemini.

Finally, Estech (San Ramon, CA) offers two bipolar clamps (one reusable and another single use), both called the Cobra Bipolar Clamp.

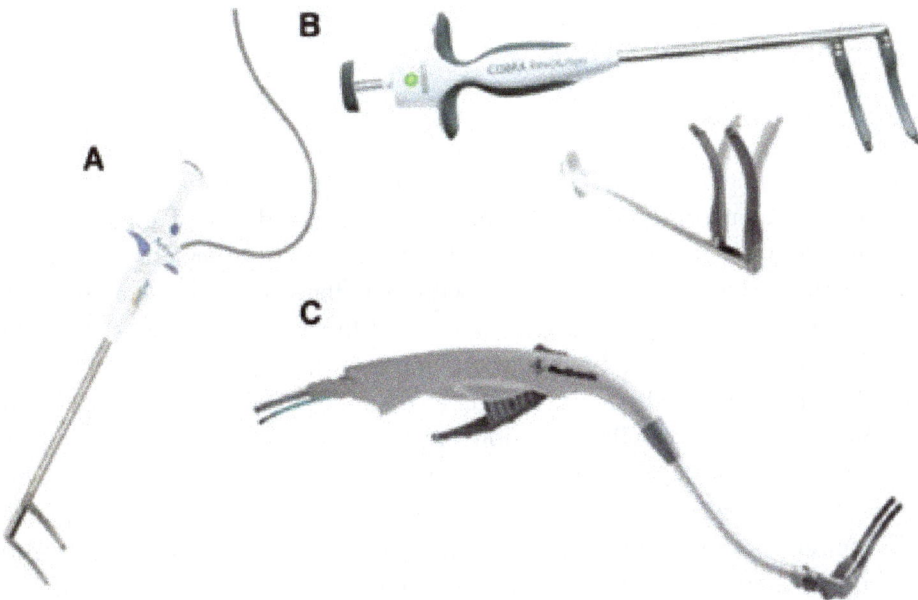

Figure 5. Available devices for bipolar RF ablation.

In bipolar devices, alternating current is generated between two closely approximated electrodes. This results in a more focused ablation than with unipolar technology. As for unipolar technology, ablation occurs by resistive heating, but, as the energy passes between the two electrodes, temperatures reach 60–70°C between the electrodes but drops off quickly in neighboring tissue. Bipolar RF ablation results in discrete, transmural lesions, with no evidence of contraction or scarring.

In an animal model using bipolar clamps, microscopic examination showed that 99–100% of all lesions were transmural, continuous, and discrete with a single ablation using the conductance algorithm. Bipolar clamps are the fastest and most reliable devices for creating transmural lesions in open procedures, both on the beating and the arrested heart, with average ablation times between 5 and 10 s [13]. Compared to cryoablation, which can also effectively create transmural lesions when used for adequate time (2.5–3 min), bipolar RF use is faster. Pen devices can be effective but must be used with caution. The Isolator pen has been shown to be reliable in creating transmural lesions in tissue up to 8 mm in thickness. In several studies, the Coolrail linear pen created transmural lesions only 80% of the time with a single application of the devices, but it is reasonable to speculate that multiple applications may improve performance. With all RF devices, most non-transmural lesions occur at the ends of the line of ablation. Therefore, it is important to overlap the lesions when making an extended linear lesion to insure transmurality.

The more fearsome complication of unipolar RF (esophageal perforation) has been ward off by bipolar clamps, because, since energy application is between the jaws, extensive radiation of heat is impossible, thus preventing penetrating lesions of surrounding tissues. Nevertheless, side-by-side devices safety has not been still deeply evaluated.

The risk of creating pulmonary veins stenosis especially in case of multiple and repeated RF or cryothermal lesion lines theoretically exists, but only anecdotal cases have been presented in medical literature.

2.4. Treatment of concomitant AF

2.4.1. Indications and exclusion criteria

The Heart Rhythm Society Task Force on Catheter and Surgical Ablation of Atrial Fibrillation (2012) released an expert consensus statement that included indications for surgical AF ablation [14]. They recommended that surgical ablation should be considered as an additional procedure in all patients with symptomatic AF, with or without trial of antiarrhythmic drugs, in cases where these patients were already scheduled to undergo cardiac surgery for other indications. This represents a class IIa indication for paroxysmal, persistent, and long-standing persistent AF failing antiarrhythmic drugs and paroxysmal and persistent AF prior to a trial of antiarrhythmic drugs. It is a class IIb indication for long-standing persistent AF prior to a trial of antiarrhythmic drugs. In 2016, the European Society of Cardiology (ESC), in collaboration with the European Association for Cardiothoracic Surgery, released guidelines for the management of AF [15]. Concerning fibrillating patients undergoing cardiac surgery, they recommended that maze surgery should be considered in symptomatic patients with AF (class IIa) and may be considered in asymptomatic patients in AF (class IIb). The ESC AF guidelines also proposed that AF surgery and extensive ablations should be discussed by an "Atrial Fibrillation Heart Team" comprising a cardiologist with expertise in antiarrhythmic drug therapy, an interventional electrophysiologist, and a cardiac surgeon with expertise in AF surgery.

All these recommendations assume that both the patient and the surgery meet the necessary requirements for procedural success: suitable atrial anatomy (left atrial dimensions and fibrosis), AF time of evolution, favorable risk/benefit relation, and operator experience. More in detail, the main factors associated with scarce success rate of maze, thus representing a contraindication to the procedure, are [16] advanced patient's age (but no real cutoff has been identified), left atrial size superior to 60 mm or 135 ml/mq, and an arrhythmia duration longer than 60 months. All these features arise from different trials but do not play an uncontested and universally accepted role, even if it is reasonable to hypothesize that they well correlate with AF chronicity, which translates into more deeper pathophysiological changes in the left atrium rendering arrhythmia interruption more difficult.

2.4.2. General surgical principles

Many surgical variations concerning lesions sets have been proposed, ranging from the simple isolation of the pulmonary veins (PVI) to the complete biatrial approach originally described by Cox; all types of energy sources have been tested over time too. It is difficult to indicate what is the right approach for every AF category, because studies comparing the different maze variations are scarce and most frequently do not comprise large number of patients. The result is that no unanimous consensus exists and that the task of assessing if any of lesions sets or techniques is more effective is a real challenge. Nevertheless, thanks to our knowledge concerning AF pathophysiology, we can perhaps affirm that in case of paroxysmal arrhythmia not associated to mitral disease (where we may imagine that focal triggers around pulmonary veins origin play a major role in the absence of left atrial enlargement and histologic modifications leading to reentrant drivers perpetuating circuits), a simple procedure of PVI could be sufficient. On the contrary, when the patient is affected by persistent or permanent AF, a more extensive lesions set including left atrial Cox-maze IV lines (**Figure 6**) and, if possible, right atrial ablations seems to be the best option. In fact, such a wide approach should allow the highest chances of interrupting rotors maintaining arrhythmia. The same ablation protocol may also be applied if the principal pathology requiring surgery is a mitral disease, independently from AF type: as a matter of fact, mitral valve dysfunction (stenosis or regurgitation) causes left atrial dilatation, microscopic modifications, and fibrosis which constitute a perfect substrate for arrhythmia perpetuation, thus suggesting the opportunity of a more aggressive ablation treatment. An algorithm showing how the type of AF and the extension of the structural disease may affect the type of lesions set is presented in **Figure 7** [4].

2.4.3. Outcomes

Published reports of surgical ablation contain success rates of 60–90% [1]. Factors related to the probability of success include AF duration, left atrial size, patient's age, and adaptation of lesions set to arrhythmia type and underlying disease [16]. In case of Cox-maze IV lesions set application (for instance, for mitral patients or chronic AF), completed either with cryothermy or a combination of RF and cryothermy, 1-year and longer-term freedom from AF generally range from 65 to 85%; freedom from AF off antiarrhythmic drugs tends to be about 10% lower. Success rate dramatically drops if PVI alone is performed with persistent or long-standing persistent AF with a failure percentage joining nearly 80% of the time. Patients and surgeons must understand that

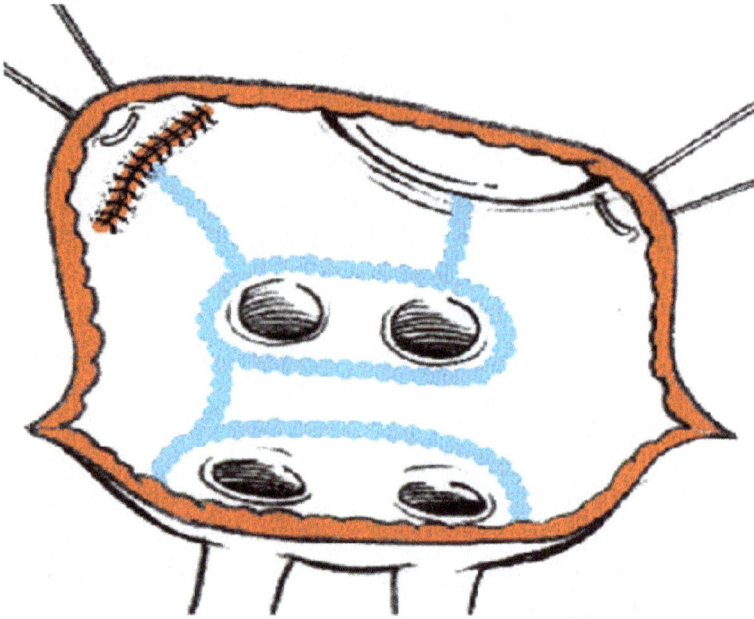

Figure 6. Modified left atrial Cox-maze IV.

the success of surgical ablation cannot be determined at the index hospitalization. During the first 6 months after surgery, half or more of patients experience atrial arrhythmias. One-year success is determined by a long-term Holter monitor (24 h or greater), confirming freedom from any episode of AF, atrial flutter, or atrial tachycardia that lasts more than 30 s. ECG alone overestimates the success by 10–15% when compared with long-term monitoring. According to guidelines, "true" success requires that the patient has no atrial arrhythmias and be off antiarrhythmic drugs. In practice, freedom from AF on antiarrhythmic drugs often represents a good clinical result. Annual follow-up with a Holter or other long-term monitor is necessary, as AF may recur overtime.

2.4.4. Perioperative management

The two key management issues are heart rhythm and anticoagulation [1]. In the absence of evidence-based guidelines, clinical practice in these areas varies considerably. Because the Cox-maze IV does not immediately "cure" AF in most patients, both heart rhythm surveillance and management are necessary. Perioperative arrhythmia relapse occurs in at least half of all patients undergoing surgical ablation. The precise cause of perioperative AF is unknown, although changes in adrenergic tone and inflammation may contribute; these physiological conditions tend to subside with time. Preoperative β-blockers should be continued in all patients who do not have a contraindication. Anti-arrhythmic medications (more often amiodarone) may be administered as prophylaxis to all patients or only in case of new AF episodes, which must be aggressively treated by electric cardioversion if chemical one fails. Antiarrhythmic treatment should be maintained at least for 2 months after hospital discharge and then stopped in the absence of detected arrhythmia episodes; otherwise, it should be continued or restarted. Considering general maze success rate, about 20% of patients will have AF at 1-year mark: if antiarrhythmic medication has failed and symptoms persist, catheter ablation may be proposed with good outcomes. Concerning anticoagulation, as more than 50% of patients experience perioperative

AF after maze, warfarin should be continued for several months after the intervention. It is reasonable to discontinue such treatment if, at 6-months check, no AF episodes have been detected with a 24-h periodical Holter monitor, atrial contractility is fully restored at transthoracic echocardiography, LAA is well controlled, and no other indication for anticoagulation exists. Although some suggest that this decision should depend on the CHADS2 score, recent data advocate that it cannot be applied to the surgical patient. The effective LAA exclusion "per se" does not allow safe warfarin interruption, since the risk of stroke is reduced but not eliminated (two to four events per 1000 patient years) after a Cox-maze IV procedure.

2.4.5. Clinical benefits and risks of maze

It is commonly accepted that, by one side, AF presence in cardiac surgery patients is associated with increased risks of death and stroke in follow-up and, by the other, that freedom from symptomatic AF and warfarin taking (objectives frequently achieved by maze) represents important advantages. Nevertheless, there is no conclusive proof—a randomized, controlled

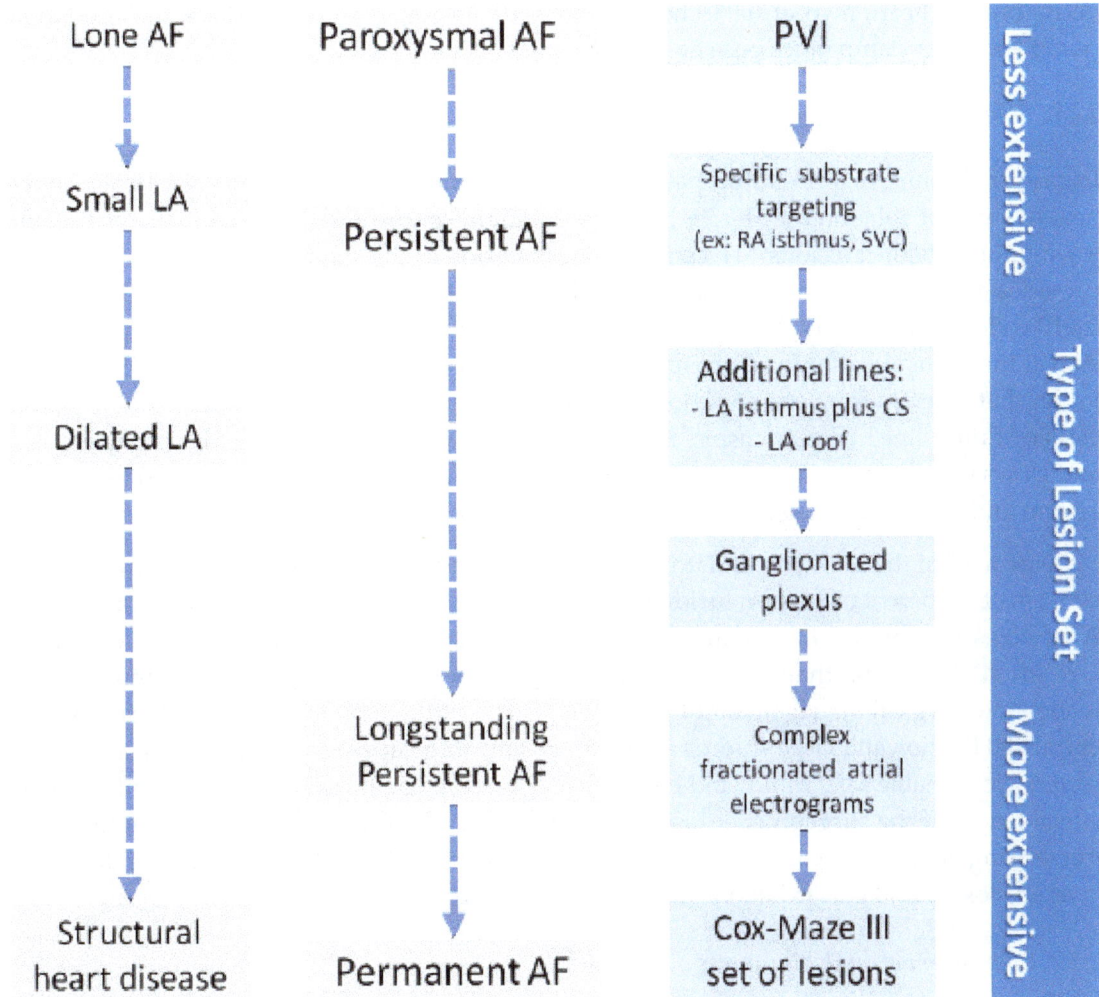

Figure 7. AF type, structural disease and lesions sets.

clinical trial—confirming that the surgical treatment of AF reduces long-term morbidity and mortality. However, we know that a successful medical and catheter-based treatment reduces late events. Observational studies, many of which employed propensity matching, suggest that successful surgical ablation has similar effects, reducing both late mortality and risk of stroke. When taking all of the available evidences together, the International Society of Minimally Invasive Cardiothoracic Surgery (ISMICS) consensus statement concluded that concomitant ablation was indicated to increase the incidence of SR at short- and long-term follow-up (class 1, level A), improve ejection fraction and exercise tolerance (class 2a, level A), and reduce the risk of stroke and thromboembolic events and improve long-term survival (class 2a, level B) [17].

In general, the addition of a Cox-maze procedure for concomitant AF ablation does not increase surgical risk as confirmed by several clinical series [18]. In addition, recent data suggest that although approximately 5% of AF patients require a permanent pacemaker after a Cox-maze IV procedure, this does not represent an increase over the pacemaker implantation rate when AF is left untreated. Finally, the surgical ablation of AF does not increase intensive care unit or hospital length of stay. Using alternate energy sources, surgical maze adds 20–25 min to the cardiopulmonary bypass time; moreover, if right atrial and PVI lesions are performed on the beating, decompressed heart, myocardial ischemic time is minimized. For most patients, the additional pump and cross-clamp times pose no supplementary clinical risk.

2.4.6. Debated issues: RA ablation and LAA management

In case of chronic AF or in mitral patients, the addition of RA lesions increases the effectiveness of surgical ablation by 10–15% [19]. The standard set proposed by Cox includes the following three distinct lesions: (1) a small (1-cm) incision in the right atrial appendage, which provides access for the creation of a cryolesion to the tricuspid annulus (tricuspid lesion at the 10-o'clock position); (2) an incision in the RA body that terminates with a second cryolesion at the tricuspid annulus (tricuspid lesion at the 2-o'clock position); and (3) an intercaval lesion that extends from the superior vena cava to the inferior one. It is a mistake to add a classic "flutter line" (cavotricuspid isthmus ablation) to this lesion set, as it is unnecessary and slows intra-atrial conduction. Creation of the standard RA lesions requires no more than 10 min and can be completed with the heart arrested or beating on cardiopulmonary bypass.

Management of the LAA is mandatory [1]. A recent prospective, randomized controlled trial confirms that percutaneous occlusion of the LAA reduces the risk of stroke in patients with AF. Successful surgical LAA management requires its complete excision or exclusion with a residual stump less than 1 cm in length [20]. Surprisingly, several studies demonstrate inadequate surgical management of the LAA, with residual flow after both endocardial and epicardial ligation and large stumps after stapled and surgical excision. New epicardial occlusion devices enable safe, rapid, and complete LAA exclusion; prospective trials confirm their effectiveness. If the surgeon chooses to use suture to exclude the LAA, a single endocardial pursestring or epicardial loop is inadequate. Endocardial exclusion should incorporate a two-layered closure and epicardial one at least two sutures.

2.4.7. Comparison of available sources

Nowadays, only RF and cryothermy remain as available sources and are currently used in medical practice separately or in combination with a similar success rate. Due to the possibility of associating different lesion line sets in different patients' category performed with unipolar, bipolar RF, or cryothermy according to surgeon's preference and habits, there is a lack of randomized-prospective trials really comparing the performance of these two technologies which are thus both accepted and employed in concomitant AF ablation.

2.5. Treatment of stand-alone AF

2.5.1. Indications

The Heart Rhythm Society Task Force on Catheter and Surgical Ablation of Atrial Fibrillation (2012) recommend that surgical ablation may be considered as a stand-alone procedure in patients who have failed antiarrhythmic drugs and who have either failed catheter ablation or who prefer surgery over catheter ablation (class IIb indication) [14]. Stand-alone surgical ablation in patients who have not trialed antiarrhythmic drugs represents a class III indication [14]. ESC guidelines (2016) [15] report that catheter or surgical ablation should be considered for symptomatic control in all cases of persistent or long-standing persistent AF that is refractory to antiarrhythmic drugs (class IIa indication). They also recommend that minimally invasive PVI should be contemplated where catheter ablation failed in symptomatic AF and that maze surgery should be considered in refractory symptomatic AF or post ablation AF to reduce symptoms (class IIa indications).

2.5.2. Minimally invasive surgical techniques and the hybrid approach

Although surgical ablation for AF is much less frequently performed as a stand-alone procedure compared to its use as a concomitant procedure, the initial report of the Cox-maze procedure was as a stand-alone procedure and was successful in providing freedom from AF in all 22 patients at 3 months [14]. The open sternotomy, "cut-and-sew" Cox-maze III procedure, has been used as a stand-alone procedure for the treatment of AF in some centers, with reports showing a success rate of 95.9% at long-term follow-up with no significant difference when compared to Cox-maze III as concomitant procedure (97.5%). Nevertheless, maze represents a very invasive operation requiring median sternotomy and, also in experienced hands, 45–60 min of cardiopulmonary bypass and cardiac arrest; as a result, efforts have been made to reduce the operative aggression in parallel with the introduction of alternative energy sources for ablation, reducing the need for "cut-and-sew" incisions. Such an approach led to the development of minimally invasive AF surgery [14, 21]. Two main operative techniques have been described:

1. A bilateral thoracoscopic approach consisting in a video-assisted bilateral mini-thoracotomy or thoracoscopic pulmonary veins island creation and LAA removal or exclusion, usually with ganglionic plexus evaluation and destruction. A monolateral approach is also possible but is technically more demanding since the device must encircle the pulmonary veins in one time passing through the transverse and the oblique sinus.

2. A right-side thoracoscopic approach with two or three ports, presenting the limitation of the inability to remove the LAA.

Nevertheless, results of mini-invasive epicardial surgical ablation were below expectations, above all when compared with those of open Cox-maze IV and cut-and-sew maze. More in detail, this was particularly true in case of non-paroxysmal AF, with a rate of freedom from arrhythmia recurrence equal to 43% for long-standing persistent AF patients. A recent systematic review estimated a 10–20% higher rate of recurrent atrial arrhythmias after minimally invasive surgery as compared to open ablation-based surgery. Based on these findings, the attention of cardiac surgeons and of cardiologists focused onto the comprehension of the reasons of such failure and, thanks to careful electrophysiological observations, highlighted that often transmurality was not achieved by current ablation tools applied endoscopically on the epicardium of the beating heart.

To overcome these limitations of minimally invasive surgical ablation as a stand-alone procedure in abolishing AF, hybrid ablation was developed, incorporating an adjunctive percutaneous catheter procedure to bridge conduction gaps in the anatomically based surgical ablation lines as well as additional targets determined electrophysiologically [22]. As a result, respective advantages and limitations were overcome and combined, allowing a relevant technical innovation.

The concept of "hybrid" procedure was first published by Pak et al. [23] who combined percutaneous epicardial catheter ablation and endocardial ablation in difficult cases of AF. According to this initial experience, other groups published their encouraging results (early freedom from AF superior to 80%) with various hybrid techniques. Actually, three different techniques are employed, each utilizing unique RF ablation tools (**Figure 8**) [21]:

1. bilateral thoracoscopy with circumferential and linear lesions (LAMP [La Meir, Ailawadi, Mahapatra, Pison] hybrid ablation) created using bipolar RF clamps and ablation pens (Atricure, West Chester, OH), respectively;

2. right-sided thoracoscopy with simultaneous isolation of PV and posterior left atrium using a suction monopolar RF catheter (Estech Cobra Adhere XL, Atricure, West Chester, OH) designed to deliver an encircling linear lesion;

3. Subxiphoid posterior pericardioscopy (through laparoscopic incision of the central diaphragmatic tendon) with linear ablation using a vacuum irrigated unipolar RF device (Numeris guided coagulation system with VisiTrax, nContact surgical, Inc., Morrisville, NC, USA) to isolate or debulk the posterior left atrium and partially isolate the pulmonary veins

PVI was a common end point in all studies. In addition to the differences in epicardial lesions created by these very different strategies and tools, the timing of the endovascular catheter component also varied widely, from being performed immediately after surgery or after a delay ranging from 4 days to 3 months. Potential advantages of the "immediate staged" strategy compared to the "delayed staged" one are (1) there is no risk of tamponade during the trans-septal puncture since the pericardium is open; (2) the surgeon can protect the phrenic nerves and the esophagus and the effective surgical ablation reduces the fluoroscopy time; (3) thromboembolic events rate consequent to endocardial ablation is reduced since the majority of lesions lines are performed epicardially.

Nevertheless, the hybrid procedure is time-consuming and the need of heparinization after septal puncture just following the "surgery time" may cause major bleeding of dissected areas.

The endovascular component itself varied significantly between studies, such as whether electroanatomical mapping was utilized, the choice of linear ablation lesions, and which patients these were performed in, whether physiological targets such as triggers and complex fractionated atrial electrograms were targeted and selection of end points including intraprocedural confirmation of conduction block and re-induction protocols. Many other aspects greatly varied among the different approaches, such as ganglion, LAA, and ligament of Marshall management and peri-procedural medical treatment. Such diversity in approach is not surprising given the relative infancy of minimally invasive surgical AF ablation and the novel ablation tools used, as well as lack of consensus within the ablation community itself on optimal strategies for persistent and long-standing persistent AF.

2.5.3. Outcomes of the hybrid approach

Published success rates from hybrid ablation, defined as maintained SR off antiarrhythmic medications at 12 months, are 74.3% overall (76.9% for paroxysmal and 73.4% for persistent/long-standing persistent AF patients) [21, 22]. The three described techniques failed to achieve the same results in terms of freedom from AF recurrence, with the LAMP approach showing

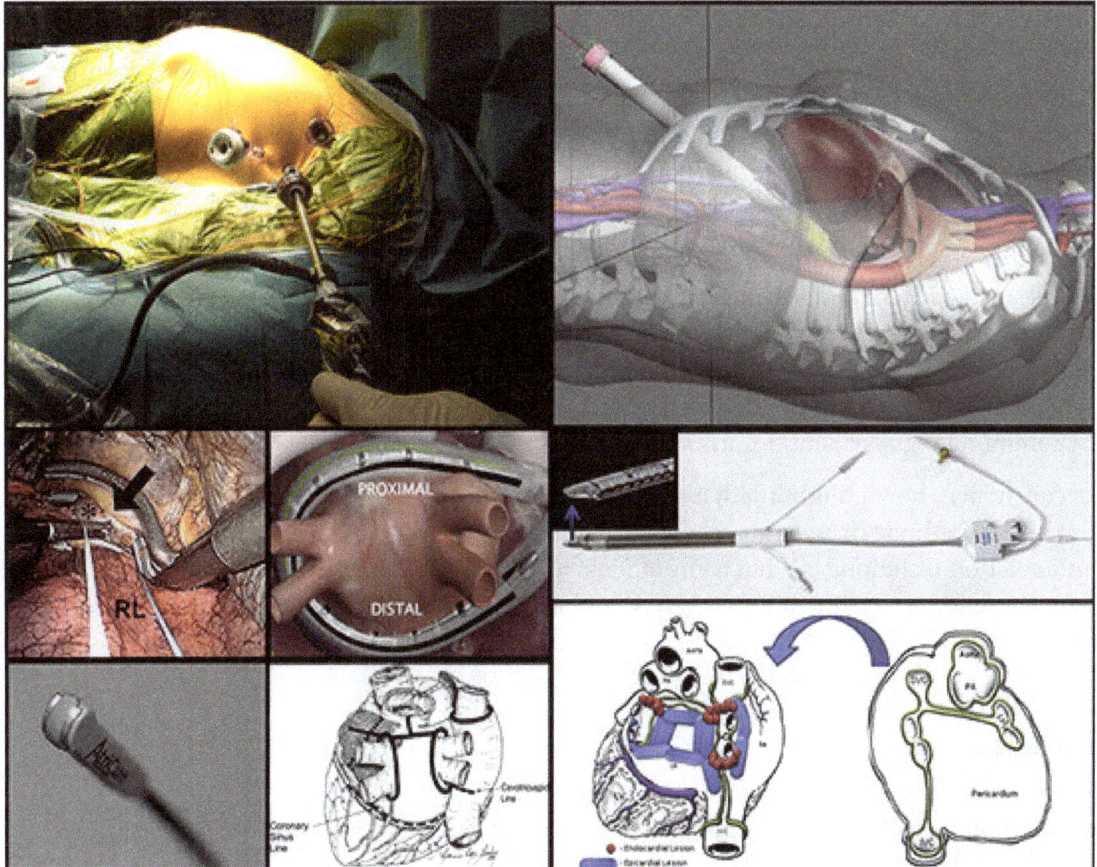

Figure 8. Hybrid ablation: access, tools and lesions sets.

the best performance (88%) and the subxiphoid posterior pericardioscopy the worst (59.3%). Even the percentage of death or non-fatal complications greatly varied from 8.5% of the bilateral approach to 0% right-sided thoracoscopy. The average length of hospital stay was between 3.6 and 7 days. A limited number of trials comparing the hybrid procedure versus sequential catheter ablation are available, but hybrid results seem to be superior than the endovascular alone ones, but with increased complications rate and longer post-procedural hospital stay.

3. Conclusions

The aim of the present treatise is to show that, thanks to the evolution in arrhythmia pathophysiology understanding, it has been possible to develop a series of different technological tools and options able to treat even long-standing persistent lone or concomitant AF, permitting a tailored procedural offer to every single patient including pure endocardial ablation, pure surgical procedures (especially for concomitant cases), or a cooperation of both (hybrid strategies).

Undoubtedly, the way is still long, since several aspects of the treatment require improvements: concerning concomitant chronic AF, first of all, rate success should be augmented by trying to develop energy sources and technologies able to achieve transmurality in the totality of cases; secondly, it should be important to join an unanimous consensus onto lesions set schema to apply, but such objective cannot be independent from a full comprehension of arrhythmia pathogenesis.

Even with reference to lone AF, understanding arrhythmia mechanisms is crucial in view of developing less invasive techniques [21]. More in detail, recent studies are now more focused on the role of autonomic ganglia in being the true triggers and perpetuators of AF and perhaps they will rapidly become the main target of future ablation techniques.

Furthermore, results of the hybrid approach are encouraging but far from perfect, especially in case of persistent and long-standing persistent AF and need to be confirmed in larger and stronger trials also allowing comparison with last-generation catheter-based ablation tools. Nevertheless, we can speculate that the success rate in the treatment of lone AF may probably rely on a close collaboration between surgeons and electrophysiologists, implying the use of "a common language" and information exchange.

In conclusion, by highlighting that midterm success results in terms of SR maintenance without antiarrhythmic drugs are satisfactory, ranging from 60 to 90% depending from AF type and ablation technique, such a comprehensive essay would like to represent a useful instrument for clinicians, allowing them to hypothesize and recommend an adapted treatment to their fibrillating patients.

Author details

Claudia M. Loardi*, Marco Zanobini and Francesco Alamanni

*Address all correspondence to: cloardi@yahoo.it

Department of Cardiac Surgery, Centro Cardiologico Monzino IRCCS, University of Milan, Milano, Italy

References

[1] Gillinov M, Soltesz E. Surgical treatment of atrial fibrillation: Today's questions and answers. Seminars in Thoracic and Cardiovascular Surgery. 2013;**25**:197-205

[2] Ad N, Suri RM, Gammie JS, et al. Surgical ablations of atrial trends and outcomes in North America. The Journal of Thoracic and Cardiovascular Surgery. 2012;**144**:1051-1060

[3] Cox J, Boineau J, Schuessler R, et al. Electrophysiologic basis, surgical development and clinical results of the maze procedure for atrial flutter and atrial fibrillation. In: Karp RB, Wechsler AS, editors. Advances in Cardiac Surgery. Vol. 6. St Louis: Mosby-Year book; 1995. p. 1

[4] Providencia R, Barra S, Pinto C, et al. Surgery for atrial fibrillation: Selecting the procedure for the patient. Journal of Atrial Fibrillation. 2013;**6**:130-138

[5] Damiano R, Gaynor SL, Bailey M, et al. The long-term outcome of patients with coronary disease and atrial fibrillation undergoing the Cox-Maze procedure. The Journal of Thoracic and Cardiovascular Surgery. 2003;**126**:2016-2021

[6] Haissaguerre M, Jais P, Shah DC, et al. Spontaneous initiation of atrial fibrillation by ectopic beats originating in the pulmonary veins. The New England Journal of Medicine. 1998;**339**:659-666

[7] Schmitt C, Ndrepepa G, Webwe S, et al. Biatrial multisite mapping of atrial premature complexes triggering onset of atrial fibrillation. The American Journal of Cardiology. 2002;**89**:1381-1387

[8] Cox J, Jaquiss R, Schuesser R, et al. Modifications of the maze procedure for atrial flutter and atrial fibrillation. Rationale and surgical results. The Journal of Thoracic and Cardiovascular Surgery. 1995;**110**:485-495

[9] Melby S, Schuessler R, Damiano R. Ablation technology for the surgical treatment of atrial fibrillation. ASAIO Journal. 2013;**59**:461-468

[10] Pan NH, Tsao HM, Chang NC, et al. Aging dilates atrium and pulmonary veins: Implications for the genesis of atrial fibrillation. Chest. 2008;**133**:190-196

[11] Lustgarden TL, Keane D, Ruskin J. Cryothermal ablation: Mechanism of tissue injury and current experience in the treatment of tachtaarrhythmias. Progress in Cardiovascular Diseases. 1999;**41**:481-498

[12] Khargi K, Deneke T, Haardt H, et al. Saline-irrigated, colled-tip radiofrequency ablation is an effective technique to perform the maze procedure. The Annals of Thoracic Surgery. 2001;**72**:S1090-S1095

[13] Melby SJ, Gaynor SL, Lubahn JG, et al. Efficacy and safety of right and left atrial ablations on the beating heart with irrigated bipolar radiofrequency energy: A long-term animal study. The Journal of Thoracic and Cardiovascular Surgery. 2006;**132**:853-860

[14] Davies R, Kumar S, Chard R, et al. Surgical and hybrid ablation of atrial fibrillation. Heart, Lung & Circulation. 2017;**26**:960-966

[15] Kirchhof P, Benussi S, Kotecha D, et al. ESC guidelines for the management of atrial fibrillation developed in collaboration with EACTS. European Heart Journal. 2016;**37**:2893-2962

[16] Gaynor SL, Schuessler RB, Bailey MS, et al. Surgical treatment of atrial fibrillation: Predictors of late recurrence. The Journal of Thoracic and Cardiovascular Surgery. 2005;**129**:104-111

[17] Ad N, Cheng DCH, Martin J, et al. Surgical ablation for atrial fibrillation in cardiac surgery: A consensus statement of the International Society of Minimally Invasive Cardiothoracic Surgery (ISMIC) 2009. Innovations. 2010;**5**:74-83

[18] Ad N, Henry L, Hunt S, et al. Do we increase the operative risk by adding the cox-maze III procedure to aortic valve replacement and coronary artery bypass surgery? The Journal of Thoracic and Cardiovascular Surgery. 2012;**143**:936-944

[19] Barnett SD, Ad N. Surgical ablation as treatment for the elimination of atrial fibrillation: A meta-analysis. The Journal of Thoracic and Cardiovascular Surgery. 2006;**131**:1029-1035

[20] Kanderian AS, Gillinov AM, Patterson GB, et al. Success of surgical left atrial appendage closure (assessment by transesophageal echocardiography). Journal of the American College of Cardiology. 2008;**52**:924-929

[21] Gelsomino S, La Meir M, Lucà F, et al. Treatment of lone atrial fibrillation: A look at the past, a view of the present and a glance at the future. European Journal of Cardio-Thoracic Surgery. 2012;**41**:1284-1294

[22] Syed F, Oral H. Electrophysiological perspectives on hybrid ablation of atrial fibrillation. Journal of Atrial Fibrillation. 2015;**8**:1290

[23] Pak HN, Hwang C, Lim HE, et al. Hybrid epicardial and endocardial ablation of persistent or permanent atrial fibrillation: A new approach for difficult cases. Journal of Cardiovascular Electrophysiology. 2007;**18**:917-923

Permissions

All chapters in this book were first published in CA, by InTech Open; hereby published with permission under the Creative Commons Attribution License or equivalent. Every chapter published in this book has been scrutinized by our experts. Their significance has been extensively debated. The topics covered herein carry significant findings which will fuel the growth of the discipline. They may even be implemented as practical applications or may be referred to as a beginning point for another development.

The contributors of this book come from diverse backgrounds, making this book a truly international effort. This book will bring forth new frontiers with its revolutionizing research information and detailed analysis of the nascent developments around the world.

We would like to thank all the contributing authors for lending their expertise to make the book truly unique. They have played a crucial role in the development of this book. Without their invaluable contributions this book wouldn't have been possible. They have made vital efforts to compile up to date information on the varied aspects of this subject to make this book a valuable addition to the collection of many professionals and students.

This book was conceptualized with the vision of imparting up-to-date information and advanced data in this field. To ensure the same, a matchless editorial board was set up. Every individual on the board went through rigorous rounds of assessment to prove their worth. After which they invested a large part of their time researching and compiling the most relevant data for our readers.

The editorial board has been involved in producing this book since its inception. They have spent rigorous hours researching and exploring the diverse topics which have resulted in the successful publishing of this book. They have passed on their knowledge of decades through this book. To expedite this challenging task, the publisher supported the team at every step. A small team of assistant editors was also appointed to further simplify the editing procedure and attain best results for the readers.

Apart from the editorial board, the designing team has also invested a significant amount of their time in understanding the subject and creating the most relevant covers. They scrutinized every image to scout for the most suitable representation of the subject and create an appropriate cover for the book.

The publishing team has been an ardent support to the editorial, designing and production team. Their endless efforts to recruit the best for this project, has resulted in the accomplishment of this book. They are a veteran in the field of academics and their pool of knowledge is as vast as their experience in printing. Their expertise and guidance has proved useful at every step. Their uncompromising quality standards have made this book an exceptional effort. Their encouragement from time to time has been an inspiration for everyone.

The publisher and the editorial board hope that this book will prove to be a valuable piece of knowledge for researchers, students, practitioners and scholars across the globe.

List of Contributors

Francisco R. Breijo-Márquez
Clinical and Experimental Cardiology (on voluntary leave), East Boston Hospital Faculty of Medicine, Boston, MA, USA

Takashi Murashita
West Virginia University, Heart and Vascular Institute, Morgantown, WV, USA

Sana Ouali, Omar Guermazi, Manel Ben Halima, Selim Boudiche, Nadim Khedher, Fathia Meghaieth, Abdeljalil Farhati, Noureddine Larbi and Mohamed Sami Mourali
Cardiology Department, La Rabta Hospital, Tunis, Tunisia

Fatma Guermazi
Psychiatry Department, Hedi Chaker Hospital, Sfax, Tunisia

Virginia Mansilla, Sergio Chain Molina and Ricardo R. Corbalán
Model Heart Center, Electrophysiology Division, Laprida, San Miguel de Tucumán, Argentina

Pablo E. Tauber
Model Heart Center, Electrophysiology Division, Laprida, San Miguel de Tucumán, Argentina
ZJS Hospital Health Center, Unit of Arrhythmias and Electrophysiology, San Miguel de Tucumán, Argentina

Felix A. Albano
ZJS Hospital Health Center, Unit of Arrhythmias and Electrophysiology, San Miguel de Tucumán, Argentina

Pedro Brugada
Cardiovascular Institute, Cardiovascular Division, Free University of Brussels, UZ Brussel- VUB, Brussels, Belgium

Sara S. Sánchez and Stella M. Honoré
Department of Developmental Biology, INSIBIO (National Council for Scientific and Technical Research-National University of Tucumán), Chacabuco, San Miguel de Tucumán, Argentina

Marcelo Elizari
Emeritus FACC, National Academy of Medicine, Buenos Aires, Argentina

Federico Figueroa Castellanos
Clinica Mayo de UMCB, Unit of Arrhythmias and Electrophysiology, San Miguel de Tucumán, Argentina

Damian Alzugaray Bioeng
Abbott, Argentina

Hamid Reza Bonakdar
St. Michael Hospital, Affiliated to University of Toronto, Canada

Antoine Deliniere, Francis Bessiere, Adrien Moreau, Alexandre Janin, Gilles Millat and Philippe Chevalier
Hôpital Louis Pradel, Lyon, France

Nevra Alkanli
Department of Biophysics, Faculty of Medicine, T.C. Halic University, Istanbul, Turkey

Arzu Ay
Department of Biophysics, Faculty of Medicine, Trakya University, Edirne, Turkey

Suleyman Serdar Alkanli
Department of Biophysics, Faculty of Medicine, Istanbul University, Istanbul, Turkey

Takumi Yamada
Division of Cardiovascular Disease, University of Alabama at Birmingham, Birmingham, AL, USA

Claudia M. Loardi, Marco Zanobini and Francesco Alamanni
Department of Cardiac Surgery, Centro Cardiologico Monzino IRCCS, University of Milan, Milano, Italy

Index

A

Acute Coronary Syndrome, 30, 34-35, 71
Amphetamine, 36-37, 44
Antiarrhythmic Drug Therapy, 41, 158
Atherogenesis, 32
Atrial Dilatation, 159
Atrial Fibrillation, 5, 16-17, 21, 23-25, 27-28, 32, 34, 38-39, 42-43, 69, 71, 84-88, 98-99, 106, 123-125, 149, 158, 163, 167-168
Atrial Tachyarrhythmia, 69
Atypical Flutter, 69-72, 82

B

Benzodiazepine, 31-33, 38
Bilateral Thoracoscopy, 164
Biopsy, 46-47, 52
Bipolar Clamp, 157
Bipolar Radiofrequency Energy, 21-22, 28, 157, 167
Breijo Pattern, 1, 5-6, 9-11, 13-15
Breijo's Electrocardiographic Model, 1
Brugada Syndrome, 46-47, 62, 64-68, 88-98, 100, 102-105, 116, 124-125

C

Cardiac Arrhythmias, 1, 18-21, 26, 29-30, 34, 36, 39, 106
Cardiac Dysrhythmia, 106
Cardiac Electrical Systole, 1
Cardiac Surgery, 25, 149-150, 153, 158, 161, 166-168
Cardiomyopathy, 15, 36, 72, 91, 101, 111-113, 124, 126-127, 133, 142-143
Cardiotoxic Illicit Drug, 30
Cardioverterdefibrillator, 47
Catecholamine Excess, 30, 32, 36, 38-39
Cavotricuspid Isthmus, 69, 76, 85-86, 162
Cell Metabolism, 18
Chagasic Myocarditis, 61
Cocaine, 30-34, 36-42
Coronary Vasospasm, 31
Cox-maze Evolution, 151
Cryoablation, 16-21, 23-24, 26-27, 153-155, 158

Cryoenergy, 152-153, 155
Cryolesion, 19, 26, 162
Cryothermal Energy, 19-20, 153
Cytoplasmic Disorganization, 61

D

Diabetes Mellitus, 106-107
Differential Pacing, 69, 80-81, 87
Drug Abuse, 29-30, 35, 38, 43

E

Electrocardiography, 8, 47
Endocardial Hypothermia, 20, 27
Endocardial Necroses, 22
Endocardium, 48, 50, 58, 60, 62, 90, 97
Epicardial Fat Infiltration, 60
Epicardium, 48, 50-51, 54, 58-61, 65, 90, 94, 97, 136, 164
Epilepsy, 4, 14
Epinephrine, 32, 34, 38, 41
Extreme Hyperthermia, 31

F

Flecainide Testing, 46, 49, 53, 59

G

Gene Polymorphism, 106-124

H

Histological Transmurality, 16
Hybrid Ablation, 149, 164-165, 167-168
Hypertension, 34, 36, 106-109, 112, 115, 123

I

Idiopathic, 41, 113, 126-128, 130, 132-133, 136, 141-148
Idiopathic Ventricular Arrhythmias, 126, 145-147
Illicit Drug, 29-30, 35, 38-40, 43
Inflammatory Phase, 18-19
Isthmus Block, 69, 79-80

L

Lymphocytic Infiltration, 61
Lythemia, 2

M

Maze Procedure, 16-18, 21, 23-24, 27, 150, 162-163, 167

Methadone, 37, 39, 44

Methamphetamine, 36, 39, 44

Mortality Rate, 106, 151

Myocardial Infarction, 19, 30-33, 35, 37-39, 41-44, 70, 80, 101, 106-107

Myocardial Injury, 19

Myocardium, 19, 22-23, 26, 32, 38, 71, 97, 110, 117, 128-129, 133, 136, 154

P

Palpitations, 1-2, 7, 14, 35, 52, 71

Paroxysmal, 8, 18, 21, 27, 36, 70, 151, 158-159, 164-165

Polymorphonuclear Leukocytic Infiltrate, 19

Programmed Ventricular Stimulation, 46-47, 63, 66

Pulmonary Vein, 24-25, 27, 34, 113

Q

Quinidine Therapy, 47

R

Radiofrequency Ablation, 16, 18, 21-25, 27-28, 33, 40, 48, 59, 63, 69, 85-87, 94, 167

Radiofrequency Catheter Ablation, 27, 47, 87, 145-147

Regional Depolarization Time, 46, 56

Replacement Fibrosis Phase, 18-19

S

Septal Puncture, 164

Sinus Bradycardia, 30, 33, 35-37, 39-40, 92

Structural Heart Disease, 16, 34-35, 38, 48, 70, 87, 112, 124, 126, 142

Sudden Cardiac Death, 1, 14, 29, 32, 36, 38, 42, 47, 63-64, 100, 117

Supraventricular Tachycardia, 7-8, 32, 36, 39, 69

Syncope, 5, 7, 35, 37, 39, 43-44, 46, 48-50, 52-53, 59, 66, 90-92, 95

T

Tachycardia, 1, 7-8, 30-40, 43, 48, 63, 68-70, 72, 74-77, 85-87, 101, 105, 126-127, 133, 144-148, 150, 160

Thaw Phase, 18-19

Thoracic Discomfort, 14

Thoracoscopy, 164, 166

Thrombolysis, 32

U

Unipolar Radiofrequency Energy, 155

V

Ventricular Fibrillation, 4, 38, 48, 63, 65, 67-68, 88, 90-92, 94-100, 104-105, 130, 156

Ventricular Tachycardia, 30, 32-33, 35-36, 38-40, 43, 48, 63, 68, 105, 126, 144-148